W9-AGG-419

PRAISE FOR CATHERINE GRAY'S WRITING

'Haunting, admirable and enlightening'
The Pool

'Gray's fizzy writing succeeds in making this potentially boring-as-hell subject both engaging and highly seductive'
The Bookseller

'Like listening to your best friend teach you to be sober. Light-hearted but serious, it's packed with ideas, tools, tips and, most importantly, reasons for living a sober life. This book is excellent.'
Eric Zimmer, host of podcast The One You Feed

'Catherine's writing style and voice captivate me. She has a way of translating her story into an experience I don't want to end. I want to drink every drop she produces.'
Holly Whitaker, founder of Tempest Sobriety School and co-presenter of Home podcast

'Hard to put down! This book combines a riveting, raw yet humorous memoir with actionable and well researched advice for anyone looking for the joy of a sober lifestyle. Catherine Gray combines storytelling and science, creating a throughly readable and unexpectedly educational read. Her contribution to this genre is truly unique. Not only entertaining; it holds a universe of hope for the reader. I highly recommend this wonderful book.'
Annie Grace, author of This Naked Mind: Control Alcohol, Find Freedom, Discover Happiness & Change Your Life

'This book is great. A balanced, informative and entertaining mélange of memoir, sociology and psychology. I identified very strongly with huge sections of it.'

Jon Stewart, guitarist of Sleeper and Leaving AA, Staying Sober blogger

'Sober is too often equated with "sombre" in our culture. Gray's book turns that idea on its head. Her experience of sobriety is joyful and life-affirming. A must-read for anyone who has a nagging suspicion that alcohol may be taking away more than it's giving.'

Hilda Burke, psychotherapist and couples counsellor

'Catherine Gray really captures the FUN we can have in sobriety. This book challenges the status quo; sobriety sounds as liberating as taking a trip to the jungle. Fun and inspirational. What an important book for our time! A joy to read.'

Samantha Moyo, founder of Morning Gloryville

'This book is a gamechanger. Everyone deserves to have Catherine hold their hand as they navigate the new world of not drinking – whether exploring alcohol-free periods or going for full on sobriety – and this book enables just that. Wise, funny and so relatable, *The Unexpected Joy of Being Sober* adds colour to the "dull" presumption that often comes with not drinking. A book for the times as sobriety continues to be the "wellness trend to watch". Keep it in your bag as you navigate the world of not drinking, and let Catherine lead the way for you as she re-defines sobriety in the 21st century.'

Laurie, Girl & Tonic blogger

the
unexpected
joy of
the
ordinary

the
unexpected
joy of
the
ordinary

in celebration of being average

CATHERINE GRAY

aster

An Hachette UK Company

www.hachette.co.uk

First published in Great Britain in 2019 by Aster, an imprint of

Octopus Publishing Group Ltd

Carmelite House, 50 Victoria Embankment

London EC4Y 0DZ

www.octopusbooks.co.uk

Copyright © Catherine Gray 2019

Distributed in the US by Hachette Book Group

1290 Avenue of the Americas

4th and 5th Floors, New York, NY 10104

Distributed in Canada by Canadian Manda Group

664 Annette St, Toronto, Ontario, Canada M6S 2C8

All rights reserved. No part of this work may be reproduced or utilized in any form or by any means, electronic or mechanical, including photocopying, recording or by any information storage and retrieval system, without the prior written permission of the publisher.

Catherine Gray has asserted her right under the Copyright, Designs and Patents Act 1988 to be identified as the author of this work

ISBN 978-1-78325-337-1

A CIP catalogue record for this book is available from the British Library.

Printed and bound in the UK

10 9 8 7 6 5 4 3 2 1

Some names and identities have been changed

Publishing Director: Stephanie Jackson

Senior Editors: Pauline Bache and Sophie Elletson

Copyeditor: Caroline Blake

Art Director: Yasia Williams-Leedham

Cover Design: Luke Bird

Typesetter: Jeremy Tilston at The Oak Studio

Production: Lisa Pinnell

Research Assistant: Charlotte Bowerman

For all the ordinary, average, regular folk out there
who feel like they're failing, but who are actually *winning*

CONTENTS

ordinary *adj.* Not interesting or exceptional; commonplace.
SYNONYMS: Average, normal, run-of-the-mill, standard, typical, middle-of-the-road, common, unremarkable, unpretentious, modest, simple, homespun, workaday, humdrum, mundane, unmemorable, pedestrian, uninspiring, bland, mediocre, garden-variety, bog-standard, nothing to write home about
ANTONYMS: Unusual, extraordinary, unique, exceptional

'I just happen to like ordinary things. When I paint them, I don't try to make them extraordinary. I just try to paint them ordinary-ordinary.'

Andy Warhol

PREFACE

Let's start on a light note, shall we?

Nah, let's dive right into the deep end. This book is not going to swim in the shallows.

Back in 2013, I was suicidal because I was in constant pain. The pain was mostly psychological, but it was also physical, because where the brain goes, the body follows.

Thoughts like, 'There's a high bridge. I could jump off it. Hmmm,' had begun to pop into my head as casually as people think about what they'll have for dinner.

Suicidal ideation is not selfish, as per the Old Testament way of thinking about mental health. It's a case of the scales tipping. It's when the angst of existing starts to outweigh your fear of being blotted out. In my experience, you think your loved ones secretly hate you anyhow, so maybe they'd be better off without you.

Depression was, for me, when the odd raven in the sky was joined by more and more winged worries, dreads and dark memories, until they crowded out the sun.

A group of ravens is, very aptly, called 'an unkindness'. Suicidal thoughts are an unkindness too; you no longer feel capable of showing love for yourself and, by extension, often others too, since hurt people *hurt people*.

Yet, by early 2014 I had transmogrified into a totally different person, one who still experienced brief eclipses of hope, but mostly alit upon bright skies, and couldn't imagine ever again wanting to leave this life. I haven't had a suicidal thought, even for a millisecond, since 2013.

Why? Three beautifully simple, yet also fiendishly difficult things. First up were two immediate life decisions that stopped me from doing myself a mischief. I quit drinking* and then, because I knew the alcohol would find its way back into my hand unless I changed mentally too, I learned to locate the forgotten joy of the ordinary (which we'll talk about here).

I would later go on to dismantle my love addiction*. Getting my addictions under control was about as relaxing as putting an octopus to bed.

---

* Both of these topics – quitting drinking and my year off dating – are covered extensively in my first two books, *The Unexpected Joy of Being Sober* and *The Unexpected Joy of Being Single*, if you're at all interested.

In my quest to re-enchant the everyday, I learned to see the 'Kindness is free, hate is expensive' gold marker graffiti outside the newsagent. To see the seam of beauty that runs through suburban pastorals, from the overly pruned garden with a gaggle of gnomes, to the fierce yearly 'our Christmas lights are bigger than yours' watt-offs, as if trying to coax Blixen and Santa from outer space down to Solihull.

Being disenchanted with our ordinary lives is our default; the Times New Roman of our evolution and biology. Our brain is naturally negatively biased. It zeroes in on what's wrong with our day, and where the predators and pitfalls are, before it lands on the positive.

It's not your brain's fault; it's just trying to save your life. But, we can retrain our brains, thanks to the marvel of neuroplasticity. We'll discuss this in great depth later by talking to experts in evolution, neuroscience and psychology.

To counter my urge to drink myself into oblivion and stare at bridges, I made it my mission to learn how to be default happy, rather than default disgruntled. To be a positive-seeking searchlight, rather than a negative-seeking drone. I managed it too.

The tactics I used might work for you too…or they might not. You are you, and I am me, and we are different. This is no 'happiness guaranteed in seven days!' self-help bait and switch. In the words of Morpheus from *The Matrix*, 'I can only show you the door. You're the one that has to walk through it.'

I mean, that's a touch melodramatic, but my point is, all books do is show you doors. No book can *make you happy*, and any book that claims to be imbued with that magical quality ought to be regarded with a 'riiiight' and an arched eyebrow.

I'm no snake oil dealer. I also can't sell you a skirting board ladder, striped paint, a bucket of gas, or a bag o' sky hooks either*. All I can do is show you *how I* learned to go from suicidal to baseline-happy; I cannot promise you will experience the same.

But it's possible this book may have that side effect. I hope so.

Catherine

---

* I was once sent out to buy these imaginary items from a hardware store, by a mischievous boss. I returned empty handed and hot-cheeked with confusion, only to find my boss rolling on the floor, crying with laughter.

INTRODUCTION

Allow me to introduce you to the person I was before I gained an appreciation of the ordinary. Fair warning: she is a bit of a tosser.

I'd always desperately wanted to work on glossy women's magazines and I'd somehow manage to shoehorn my way in, aged 23. My pay was low compared to my university friends in marketing, law and accounting (I even earned less than the trainee teachers), but on the flipside I led the most charmed, gilded, extraordinary life.

I was a saucer-eyed girl plucked from South Birmingham, who felt like she'd spent the bulk of her teenage years squinting at the road and wondering where the bloody bus was.

So when I entered the magazine realm, I was as bouncy as Will Ferrell in *Elf*, and would say things like, 'Is this for me? I get to keep this?!...This canapé is life-changing...You're sending me to Bristol to write a travel article? Are you serious? HAPPY DAYS.'

I was giddy about the free, doll-sized plates at restaurant openings, the albums I gained access to before launch, the VIP lists at exclusive clubs that looked like an Arabian princess's boudoir, the Chanel make-up for £1 in the beauty sale (that was expensive, the normal brands were 50p a pop), and the dozens of free books I got sent as books editor.

I was delighted about the fact that every night I could go to a party and get a gift bag laden with posh candles, or truffles hand-rolled on the thighs of virgin goats, or facial spritzes garnished with the tears of Romanian nuns, or whateversuch thing was trending.

But as time rolled on, I did what most humans do in most lucky-duck (read: lucky-as-fuck) situations. I grew accustomed to it, and I started to pick holes, and find fault. In short, I started to want: M.O.R.E.

A few years in, I became this berk: 'I get sent too many freebies, this is ridiculous!...Why are the canapés taking so long?...I have to use my own holiday days to go to Cape Town and write a travel article, are you serious?' (I want to time-travel back, give her a slap on the calves and tell her to wise up.)

Crampons of choosiness

See, somewhere along the way I had internalized a misconception. That the way you got extraordinarily happy was by finding *what was wrong* with your current situation and therefore gaining the ability to fix it.

I thought I needed to create my own everlasting contentment by locating the faults in the current landscape and tweaking them, as if I was designing my own personalized heaven, or architecting my own district of *The Good Place*.

It meant that I was never satisfied. I would be sent to a five-star yoga retreat in Kerala (for free) to write a travel article, and yes, I would come back bragging about the wooden hut perched on the hill overlooking the Indian Ocean, and the fact that I would return from dinner to find they'd run me a bath filled with rose petals. But most of that was just intended to impress, to showboat.

Really, I spent that holiday as I always did: being a malcontent. I was unimpressed that the yoga started at 6am (so much for a holiday!) and how the only thing available for breakfast was curry (is it against their religion to fry up some bacon, for Godsake?!*). I was always wanting, striving, seeking the extraordinary, but when I was in the extraordinary, I wanted it to be *more* extraordinary.

Given I found the Keralan holiday wanting, you can imagine how I reacted to an essentially ordinary weekend of food shopping, cleaning and social commitments I didn't necessarily want to do.

My psychological state was that of the toddler who plants themself face-first on the floor of the supermarket and pounds the floor with their tiny fists, crying 'it'snotfair...Wahhhhh...lifenotfair!'

I thought people who were happy with their lot were dim nitwits who had drunk the 'this is enough' Kool-Aid, had the wool pulled over their eyes, settled for the substandard and would never reach the peaks that I would scale via the crampons of my choosiness. I had a pickaxe of pickiness and my eyes fixed on the summit, while they had a foam mallet they were happily boinging each other over the head with.

The content and thankful types stayed at home waiting for all of the missing buses that had fallen into Birmingham's version of the Bermuda Triangle. Because they were OK with ordinary, they got stuck there. I pitied the fools.

---

* Much of Kerala is Muslim. So, um, yes it is.

I wanted pots of money, a darling house with shutters, to get married at Yosemite, at least three dogs, awards on my mantlepiece, and until I got all of that, I reserved the right to be default disenchanted. I thought my discontentment with my current, imperfect, ordinary situation was what was going to power me towards my future, perfect, extraordinary situation.

And my discontentment did serve as an energy source for a while. But the problem was, as soon as I got the job/flat/person I hankered after, I would be smug for a while, but then I would tire of it, start to find faults, and flip my gaze upwards to the *next thing I wanted*.

Why we're never quite satisfied

Believe it or not, what I was experiencing has a name other than 'being an entitled fuckwit'. It's the result of something called the 'hedonic treadmill'. This treadmill is a metaphor to sum up the psychological phenomenon of 'hedonic adaptation'. Hedonic adaptation means that we adjust to our circumstances much more quickly than is desirable, and thus start searching for the next high.

It means we never reach the end of the treadmill. It continues ad infinitum. There is no 'arrival' at contented bliss. No 'you have reached your destination' ending. Because as soon as we achieve something, after a brief, fist-punching surge of euphoria, it's proven that our tendency is to snap back to the happiness we experienced *before we achieved the thing*.

And so we plateau into the post-win flatline, and proceed to leg it after the next thing. *Person runs forever*. The pursuit of happiness is freakin' tiring.

So, say we want to buy a house. We run like buggery towards it. Strive strive, pound pound, sweat sweat, and we finally make the purchase. We experience, say, six months of 'well slap me and call me Susan, I only went and *bought this house*, I own these actual walls!' *Pats wall and flicks imaginary masonry dust off shoulder*.

But then, we come down from the house-buying high. We start calculating how many of the walls we actually own (two of 'em in the living room, the bank owns the rest), and we start shooting for the next thing, whether that's a loft conversion, a promotion, a better car, a wedding ring or a baby.

Survival of the negative

On top of that, our brains are natural-born pessimists. They're like the grumpy old man in a film, typically played by Jack Nicholson.

Evolutionarily speaking, it makes sense that our brain automatically scans the horizon for potential peril. 'Survival of the negative' is more accurate than 'survival of the fittest'. There's no use in being able to run like an Olympian if you haven't spotted the thing you need to run *from*.

By homing in on what is wrong with the picture, rather than what is right with it, our brains are simply trying to save our skins, should calamity strike. It's just that now, we no longer live in landscapes where wolves or a rival tribe, or highway henchmen or the plague, threaten to eradicate us. There are threats, for sure, but if you live in the first world, you're generally pretty safe.

And yet, our brains have hung onto this ancient hardwiring, which means we survey rush hour with the same [insert air-raid siren] threat level as our ancestors would have appraised a genuinely dangerous situation. We'll talk about this much more later, with the help of experts.

The 'dis' generation

Generation X and Millennials*, more so than their parents and grandparents, have a greater tendency to be *dis*enchanted, *dis*illusioned, *dis*satisfied, *dis*gruntled...you get the picture.

One poll found that just three in ten Brits describe themselves as 'happy with their lives'. One in six of us experiences a bout of anxiety or depression at least once a week. And rates of depression worldwide increased by 18 per cent between 2005 and 2015.

I think this is because the modern condition has created all sorts of lofty expectations within us. Expectations whipped up over the waves of social media comparison, joined by a thunderclap of twenty-tens privilege, and then intensified by the gales of drug/alcohol (same thing, actually)/phone addiction. All amounting to a perfect storm of a mental health crisis.

Why do I think it's mostly a modern malaise, a young/midlife person's gig, this '*dis*' propensity? Guess who the happiest age group of people in Britain is, according to recent data gathered by the Office of National Statistics? Those aged 70 to 74 years old.

---

* We'll talk about Baby Boomers, Generation X and Millennials a lot in this book, so for the record, there are conflicting date ranges bandied about, but here's the general consensus: Baby Boomers are those born from 1944 to 1964 (those aged between 56 and 76 in 2020). Generation X were born from 1965 to 1981 (so, aged between 39 and 55 in 2020). Millennials are thus named because they 'came of age' on the millennium, so they were born from 1982 to 1996 (thus aged between 24 and 38 in 2020), and are closely followed by Generation Z.

Yep, those we would probably guess to be the least cheerful. In fact, they also sat in the eyrie of the happiness graph in 2012. Those whose joints constantly ache, who have a face full of beautiful (story)lines, whose life is mostly past tense.

And yet, they're happier than their supple, glow-cheeked, leggy-with-possibilities kids. It's crackers, but here's a big clue as to why I think this may be; the 70-ish think Facebook is called Bookface and that Twitter is 'The Twitter'. They haven't a clue. Not a blissful clue.

They only compare themselves to their immediate peers, which is comparison enough, and they don't feel as if they're in some silent competition with some pretzel-binding, backflipping yoga fiend from Santa Monica.

Mining the wonder in the workaday

After my privileged wazzock stage, I entered a deep bog of melancholy and found myself knee-deep in addiction and suicidal thoughts, so shaking off my malcontent coil became vitally important.

In recovering, I learned how to mine the wonder in the workaday. Simply by doing one thing. Writing at least five gratitudes, daily.

I nearly put myself to sleep writing that last line.

Gratitude-ing has been so done to death it's now soporific; it's become hackneyed, clichéd, blah, snore, wake me up when it's over. It was one of the most transformative daily practices I've ever adopted, and yet even I'm sick to the back teeth of articles called things like 'The Power of Gratitude'. Bore off.

We'll talk more later about why gratitude literature is so off-putting, worthy and feels like a guilt-trip for those living in the Western world. (There will be no Hail Marys or punitive chin-ups ordered here.) We'll also talk about why an 'exactitude of gratitude' rather than a vague, slippery 'attitude of gratitude' is crucial.

But for now, I discovered that if I don't let everyday pleasures slide on by unnoticed, or fall out of my head, I can get a buzz from watching Sam the Staffie swim on Brighton beach.

It may not be the same thrill as I got from watching hundreds of dolphins escorting a boat through the Indian Ocean, but once you add up a grinning dog splashing around like a seal, buttery toast, getting a seat on a packed train, a sweet conversation with a stranger – all the things that do go right in a very ordinary day – it can mean that an ordinary day begins to create the same sensation as an extraordinary day. The sum of its parts creates the same whole, or even, something greater.

My joy in the ordinary has likely made me irritating, to the gloom-mongers of the world. Former me would have hard-swerved current me. I now do things like 'ta-da!' a gifted bouquet of shower caps on Instagram with a dancing gif (life hack: use them to cover plates instead of faffing about with plastic wrap).

Whereas pre-2013, I would have been affronted by that gift from my mum. 'What the chuff is this?! Shower caps? A bouquet of *flowers* would have been more appropriate!'

I have been known to weep at the beauty of sunrises, and I want to apologize for that, because I feel deeply uncool for typing it, but I'm not going to, because positivity should not be seen as uncool. (2013-me would have hissed at 2019-me in the manner of Patsy *Absolutely Fabulous* growling at wholesome Saffy.)

The wall-to-wall ordinary

The extraordinary can bring you joy, of course. Dolphins are rad. I'm not going to pretend that I don't enjoy a luxury holiday. Hell yeah I do. Bring me that holiday. Now you can go, thxbye. *Begins to pack*

However, if you think over the past year and pluck out experiences that you would classify as 'extraordinary', how many have you got? For me, highlights include seeing a two-metre wide manta ray flap past while diving, and dining at a Michelin-starred restaurant. This means my 'extraordinary' quota is about ten days out of 365. Making the remaining 355 days, or 97 per cent of my year, 'ordinary' days.

This overwhelming and inevitable life-lean towards the ordinary is why true deep-pile contentment is found when you re-enchant the everyday. Constantly straining to put an 'extra' in front of the ordinary means that even though you may have been allocated jammy emergency exit leg room seats for free, you're eyeing up Business and First Class. Even though somebody has told you look 'nice' today, you want to be told you look gorgeous.

If you hook your happiness onto the extraordinary, you're going to find yourself kicking the dirt of disappointment, eyeing up the waterfall on the horizon. The bulk of our existence is the 'work, eat, sleep, repeat' cycle. In Britain, we spend an average of five years of our lives bored.

A tour of the ordinary

In yelling 'stranger danger!' or 'what the fuck was that?' or 'watch out for her!', our brains are just doing their jobs as our bodyguards. But that doesn't mean we can't change our brain's default setting. Neuroplasticity has lent us the power to change our cognitive autopilot. As with a 3D printer, what we input into our minds takes physical shape.

This book aims to help you take that runner off that godforsaken hedonic treadmill, allowing you to sit down and have a long look at the hill you've just belted up, at the gorgeous view you earned.

I am not an example, a role model or a self-help guru; I am just a person muddling through, who loves geeking out on psychology and neuroscience, grilling experts, deep-diving into hundreds of academic studies, trying things out and reporting back on what she's learned.

On our discovery trail of the ordinary, I'll be relentlessly pointing out humdrum things I've learned to be delighted by, and will be tirelessly, maddeningly upbeat about averageness, with about as much street-smarts and insouciance as a bouncy children's TV presenter. I warn you: I will chirp. And maybe even froth.

Then, just as you're starting to deep sigh, I will switch to being a kohl-eyed, speech-giving rejectionist of notions such as these; that we should aim to be happy 24/7, that anger is a 'bad' emotion, that capping your news consumption makes you a navel-gazer, or that we should embrace the 'always on' smartphone age.

I'll be a mildly schizophrenic kinda host. With one consistency. I'm not going to *tell you* to do anything. That's not my style. All I am is your tour guide to the underbelly of our ordinary lives.

We'll be taking in our dissatisfied neural pathways, going deep into our psychological predisposition to strive for more, and tunnelling down into the ancient evolution of our disenchantment.

The ultimate aim of this exploration? To be happy with what we already have. Who we already are. The world we currently occupy. Rather than constantly seeking to upgrade our pay packets, homes, bodies, relationships, holidays, even ourselves to [insert your name] 2.0.

Because [insert your name] 1.0 is already doing so very well.

DISCLAIMER:

I am acutely aware that I was born with a head start, having arrived yelling into the first world as white and middle-class. My viewpoint is indeed subjective and based on my lived experience, which is something I cannot change, even though I have done my damnedest to be as objective and inclusive as possible.

I wholeheartedly apologize in advance for any instances in this book where I forget to check my privilege, assume we are all able-bodied or financially level-pegging, am clumsily heteronormative, or don't stay equally weighted across genders.

'She' and 'he' are no reflection of my belief in binary gender roles as 'right', and anyone who does not feel like a 'she' or 'he' is kindly requested to supplant with 'they', or the language of their choice.

But I do hope that if you look for the similarities between us, rather than any differences, we shall locate common ground. Because all humans, once you strip it all away, are essentially the same.

With the deepest respect to all of you.

Namaste. (Yep, I'm also a yogi cliché.)

I: THE PURSUIT OF THE EXTRAORDINARY

SURVIVAL OF THE MOST NEGATIVE

Our brains collude against us, by being negative-seeking missiles.

A brilliant quote sums this up: 'The brain is like Velcro for negative experiences, but Teflon for positive ones' has now been shared millions of times.

So who better to ask why this is, than the man who said it? Enter neuropsychologist Dr Rick Hanson. The first thing he tells me is that one of the main reasons for this is that the amygdala (the brain's alarm bell) is primed to go negative in most people.

'Our brain automatically scans the environment for bad news, we over-focus on it, over-react to it, and the whole experience is prioritized in emotional memory,' Dr Hanson explains.

Fabulous.

It's why if you have a feedback review with your boss, your brain will take the one criticism they gently delivered and do this with it: spend a lot of time plucking out the exact letters, throw it up on a billboard in your brain and illuminate it in fluorescent lighting, as if it's a new film on at a retro cinema. While the positives lie on the floor, forgotten.

'LACKS CONFIDENCE' is then up in lights, while 'liked by co-workers', 'diligent' and 'polite' languish on the cutting room floor. And much like a cinema, we re-play 'LACKS CONFIDENCE' over and over.

Stone Age brains in the 21st century

But why did this negative-seeking bias evolve in the first place? 'There's a short answer for that,' says Dr Hanson, author of *Resilient: find your inner strength*. 'Carrots and sticks. We needed to get carrots and avoid sticks. Our ancestors dealt with high aggression within tribes and from predators. If they didn't spot a stick before it went "thwack!" their odds of passing on their genes nosedived.'

To unravel the conundrum further, I called on the insights of evolution expert (note: expert in my eyes, he humbly disagrees) Professor Vybarr Cregan-Reid, the author of *Primate Change: how the world we made is remaking us*.

Cregan-Reid points out that there's a mismatch between how our bodies function and the environment in which we live; essentially, our bodies haven't caught up.

'Life moves fast – evolution is slow,' is his overarching argument. Much like the pampered dog that eats and eats when it gets the chance, despite having gotten two meals a day for its entire life, primal parts of our brain don't grasp – or like – our current situation *at all*.

'Modern living is as bracing to the human body as jumping through a hole in ice,' says Cregan-Reid. Metropolises in particular freak us out. 'We think of cities as longstanding, but if the timeline for the existence of our species was thought of as a 9 to 5, even the smallest cities weren't built until well into 4.59pm. As a result, our bodies are in shock. Our limbic systems pump us full of nervous tension in response to urban environments.'

Professor Cregan-Reid cites a study performed on a building project in Chicago. The inhabitants on one side of the apartment block had access to green space, while the people in the other half had none. 'They tracked crime levels and mental health and found that the people living on the side with green space were much calmer and less likely to commit crimes.'

I tell him that my amygdala (part of the limbic system, which produces an emotional response) goes into overdrive when I step into the mayhem of busy London train stations. My Stone Age brain starts yelling and I have to talk it down using my rational prefrontal cortex.

'When you're in Euston station, you know you can access food and water on a rational level, since you've got £5 in your pocket,' says Cregan-Reid. 'Yet, your limbic system panics since it can't see any signs of life; there are no crops or water, only other humans. We're like chickens in a coop.' Ethical shoppers demand organic, free-range eggs, yet we often cram ourselves into spaces smaller than even the well-treated chickens have.

'It's your amygdala over-reacting,' explains neuroscientist Dr Alex Korb, who is the author of *The Upward Spiral: Using neuroscience to reverse the course of depression, one small change at a time*. 'That knowledge won't completely eliminate your discomfort in train stations, but it can enable you to bring your prefrontal cortex online, to remind yourself that nothing's actually wrong.'

To summarize, our jumpy amygdalas were extremely useful back in the day. They saved us from getting eaten. But now we don't need them as much. Thankfully, we also have a part of the brain that can regulate the amygdala when it wants to fight or sprint into the distance. Enter the prefrontal cortex. Often described as the 'higher' brain, it is rational, logical and according to Dr Korb, the 'adult in the room'. It's also the part of the brain which separates us from other primates, given ours is significantly larger.

Brain scans show our negative bias

Not only do our brains home in more on the negative, they also go batshit when they find it. Whereas positive things don't create the same fizz of arousal.

In a now famous study performed in 1998, called 'Negative information weighs more heavily on the brain', one of the 'founding fathers of social neuroscience' (Dr John Cacioppo, and colleagues) hooked participants up to a brain scan (an ERP) and showed them varying stimuli.

In a series of tests, they were shown three types of images; positive pictures (hilariously, a pizza, chocolate ice cream and a Ferrari, which sound like a collection of props from a scene in *Ferris Bueller's Day Off*), neutral stimuli (such as a hairdryer or a plug socket), and negative images (like a deceased cat or a gun), during which time their neural arousal was measured. The electrodes detected greater neural arousal when confronted with the negative images.

The authors of this trailblazing study also cited other 'negative bias' studies, which showed that our distress at losing a set amount of money outweighs our pleasure at gaining it.

The study also showed that, when evaluating people, negative traits are given greater weight than positive ones. So, even if you notice five positive things about a person, the negatives (mean to wait staff, wears Crocs non-ironically) are given precedence. They are literally larger in our brains.

It's even been proven that we are much faster to pick an angry face out of a crowd, than a happy one, in a phenomenon called 'the anger superiority effect'. Which is why, when you're scanning a throng of people, you will zero in on the one who could be threatening.

Our amygdala is like The Hulk

Our negatively biased 'yah, what the fuck was that?!' brains remind me of The Incredible Hulk. The Hulk is a primal, fearful, over-reacting, naïve part of us that we can't remove, but we can learn to manage.

In the 2008 incarnation of *The Incredible Hulk*, there's a scene that sums this up. Ed Norton (The Hulk) is still in his primal Hulk form. Thunder growls and lightning forks across the sky. The confused, threatened Hulk snaps off a chunk of mountain and hurls it at the storm, roaring a warning.

Liv Tyler's character Betty talks him down, telling him there's nothing to be scared of. It's just weather; not an army helicopter or the end of the world. The Hulk is our amygdala, while Betty is the prefrontal cortex.

This interplay of 'characters' in the brain is the backbone of Dr Steve Peters' million-selling *The Chimp Paradox*. We *can* use our prefrontal cortex to soothe our amygdala by constantly, gently talking it down, reminding it there's no immediate threat, and most importantly, drawing its attention to the positives instead.

Meditation is known to behave as a Betty, in mellowing and soothing a grouchy amygdala. It's a well-being cliché because it works. 'When people meditate regularly,' says Dr Hanson, 'one benefit is that their ability to regulate their amygdala with their prefrontal cortex and hippocampus increases, which could produce a calmer, less reactive amygdala.'

Why? One Harvard study discovered that just eight weeks of meditation thickened the cerebral cortex; in particular the prefrontal cortex. Interestingly, the thickening was most pronounced in the *older* participants of the study.

We *can* change our brains. Ensuring that The Hulk knows that a simple thunderstorm is just weather; not the impending apocalypse.

THE HEDONIC TREADMILL

The phrase 'hedonic treadmill' was coined by two psychologists (named Brickman and Campbell) in the 1970s to sum up a psychological phenomenon called 'hedonic adaptation'. Hedonic itself means 'connected with feelings of pleasure' and is closely related to 'hedonistic'.

Hedonic adaptation is a wildly interesting quirk that humans possess to adapt to both positive and negative experiences. Victory wears off; agony does too. Euphoria fades; despair too. Love wanes; heartbreak too. And life events that we expect to clinch eternal happiness, or spell cataclysmic lifelong doom, just...*don't*.

'We overestimate how long and how intensely a particular negative life event (such as a terminal diagnosis or being fired from a cherished job) will throw us into despair,' says Professor of Psychology, Sonja Lyubomirsky. Great! So, we bounce back more quickly than we anticipate.

However, there's a catch. This goes both ways. We also overestimate the impact of positive events too. 'How long and how intensely a particularly positive event (earning lifetime tenure or having our marriage proposal accepted) will throw us over the moon,' Professor Lyubomirsky adds.

The treadmill metaphor

Adaptation lends itself to a treadmill metaphor, because the quest for satisfaction is a neverending belt. Every buzz tends to wear off, every high swoops back down, every whoop of triumph fades, which means this: we're never quite sated. Our happiness tends to readjust to baseline, no matter what. No matter how hard you run, you never complete the race. There's always more belt to pound.

This is why, as a society, we are hypnotized by the promise of being better; like a swaying cobra or a swinging clock. It's why daytime TV is monopolized by makeover shows, showcasing the promise of a better garden, a better body, an upgraded wardrobe. We sit, enraptured, taking mental notes, watching *The World's Most Extraordinary Homes*, wanting.

Satisfaction and 'enough' is an ever-moving target. You're living with your folks, so you want to move out. Once you have a driving licence, you want a car. Once you're renting, you want to buy. Once you've got that first job, you want the next job. When you're in a relationship, you want to live together. When you live together, you want to get married.

More, more, more. Move, move, move.

In our brain, the 'hedonic hotspot' is the nucleus accumbens, and it's not a fan of the habitual, the expected or, indeed, the ordinary. It would probably douse this book in petrol and chuck a match at it.

'Our nucleus accumbens is very good at habituating to whatever our life currently is,' says Dr Korb, who has studied the brain since 2002. 'It's excited by the unexpected, the infrequent, the unusual. So, if every week you get a cheque through the post, the nucleus accumbens is bored by it. Whereas if you get an *unexpected* cheque, it releases a rush of dopamine.'

Many of the studies on hedonic adaptation look at our response to huge life events – marriage, bereavement, new baby, divorce, lottery winning – but we adapt to the minutiae of life too.

'We even adapt to a massage while it's happening,' says Professor Lyubomirsky. 'At 40 minutes in, we're not loving it as much as we did at ten minutes in,' says the author of *The Myths of Happiness: what should make you happy, but doesn't, what shouldn't make you happy, but does.*

'The first time you use Uber, you're awestruck; "this is amazing"', says Dr Korb. 'But just a couple of weeks later you've forgotten how awestruck you were, and you're displeased that you have to wait six minutes for a ride.'

How consumerism capitalizes on our hedonic treadmill

Consumerism tells us that happiness is on a Caribbean sunlounger, in the driving seat of a galloping horse-powered car, or inside an expensive golden locket. Satisfaction is available if you buy this course for just £59.99! Contentment is available from the high street. Zen could be yours today via bank transfer.

I don't buy it anymore. Do you?

Advertisers profiteer from, and deliberately peddle, our dissatisfaction. It's no coincidence that the most 'extraordinary' things are the most expensive.

Consumerism lives and dies on one thing: the desire for more. Satisfaction is the altar on which consumerism dies a gruesome death. Which means there are millions of clever people out there whose sole purpose is to convince us that we don't have enough, and that we need to upgrade, to snag, to bag, to go out and smash-grab as many goods and services as we possibly can.

It sells us the idea that happiness is at the bottom of shopping bags. There is a seductive billion-pound industry constructed around making us feel like what we currently have is grey, boring and due a <click here to upgrade today!>.

But locating the ultimate consumer satisfaction is as unattainable as finding the exact GPS spot of the end of the rainbow, and standing there bathed in its violet and buttercup rays. No matter how much you move towards the end of the rainbow, it stays the same distance away from you.

It's an optical illusion made of raindrop prisms, not a destination you can reach. Consumerism is the exact same unattainable, unreachable illusion. There is no arrival at the sweet spot of enough, no matter how much we buy.

We can't get no satisfaction

They tell us that spending money makes us happy, in a bajillion different ways. OK, thanks for that adverts.

But then, why-oh-why do those of us who spend more of a percentage of our income, show 'lower global satisfaction' as happiness/spending analyst Ed Diener reports? Spending is a feathered, flashing thing glinting in the water, that we lunge for, only to find we have been hooked into a trap.

Buying things is thrilling upon the point of purchase, but quickly wears off.

'The glory of acquisition starts to dim with use, eventually changing to boredom as the item no longer elicits even a bit of excitement,' says the Japanese minimalist, Fumio Sasaki.

'This is the pattern of everything in our lives,' he continues. 'No matter how much we wish for something, over time it becomes a normal part of our lives, and then a tired old item that bores us, even though we did actually get our wish. And we end up being unhappy.'

Big splurges are actually counter-productive. Research has found that we're better dividing up any spending money we have into small, regular portions. 'Think frequent, rather than intense,' says Professor Lyubomirsky.

Campaign message: you are not enough

Even more sinister, is the way that the behemoths sell to us, by subtly telling us that where we are is not good enough, or our lives are sub-par, and dangling the carrot of satisfaction perpetually out of crunching range.

The lynchpin of consumerism – the tacks that hold the entire system together – is this message: you need to change what you are / what you look like / what you have / what you put into your body. And social media has provided a really handy 'keep up with the Kardashians' vehicle.

The regional differences in what is upheld as the ideal, show how ugly the subtext of consumerism can be. When I was in the Philippines visiting my stepmother and late father, I saw an appalling skin-lightening advert whereby a Filipino model was unzipping her beautiful golden face to reveal a lily-white one beneath.

I came home to see, of course, self-tanning adverts that encouraged the exact opposite transition. For us to look as if we're from Spain, when we're really not.

Whatever we don't naturally have, we are told we need. It's why my Filipino stepmother was constantly baffled by my dedication to sunbathing each day on that trip, while she determinedly kept out of the sun. We have been marketed into wanting each other's shade of skin.

Are kids wired to seek out the extraordinary?

Me, pointing to a low-flying seagull, exposing its downy, white, fattened-by-seaside-chips belly. 'I like seagulls.'

Five-year-old Charlotte glances and sighs. 'I like leopards.'

Is disenchantment nature or nurture? Are we created with a satisfaction-shaped hole, or is it human-made?

I conducted a totally unscientific and entirely unrepresentative study of a couple of dozen kids I know, and discovered that the age when kids stop being filled with The Wonder, and start being possessed by 'I want!' instead, is age four or five, when they go to school. A coincidence, or the fact they are starting to be exposed to social norms, oneupmanship, and keeping up with the Chloes and Georges?

Their enchantment seems to drain from them the moment they set foot in a playground and start seeing other people's backpacks, lunch boxes, scooters, coats, shoes, parents. They develop a 'where's mine?' reflex upon hearing tales of slides, gadgets and gargantuan toys.

'I love the painted cardboard box in our garden that serves as a makeshift boat' becomes 'Why don't we have a trampoline, Mummy?'

We're not born consumers, I don't think, but we are Play-Doh-ed into them, and very early on. My niece and nephew went through a phase of manically clicking on those YouTube videos that show other kids opening presents.

If you didn't know about this, it's a real thing. Kids are now huge YouTube stars for doing toy reviews. The top cat is an eight-year-old, LA-based kid called Ryan, who has 20 million followers, and whose 'Christmas morning 2016' post has been watched 114 million times. Oosh.

I mean, I can hardly talk. My first word was 'mine'. And when I was four, my favourite book was probably the toy section of the Argos catalogue.

Overriding the hedonic treadmill

Hedonic adaptation is often presented as a fait accompli, but there are ways to hoodwink hedonic adaptation. To prolong pleasure. And stop buzzes from wearing off.

'Say if you have a favourite tea,' says Professor Lyubomirsky. 'If you drink it all the time, it will lose its effect. So try not to do it too often. But I think many of us know this intuitively.' I tell her I definitely don't, and if I like something I do it *all the blinkin' time*. She laughs.

Interrupting the activity also increases the hedonic pleasure, strangely enough. 'People enjoy massages more when they are interrupted with a 20-minute break, enjoy television programmes more when they are interrupted with commercials and enjoy songs they like more when they are interrupted with a 20-second gap,' says Professor Lyubomirsky.

Dr Hanson sent me an illuminating paper that seeks to overturn the idea that the hedonic treadmill is inevitable ('Beyond the Hedonic Treadmill: revising the adaptation theory of well-being').

The expert authors of this paper believe the hedonic treadmill can be overridden, and that our set points of happiness can be improved and raised, long-term. 'Adaptation is a powerful force, but it is not so complete and automatic that it will defeat all efforts to change well-being,' the authors wrote.

The paper presents powerful evidence that random acts of kindness and gratitude practices elevate well-being, big time. This 'contradicts the idea of an unchangeable baseline for happiness,' the paper reports.

There should be an extra emphasis on 'random', says Professor Lyubomirsky. At the University of California, she and her students tested this out. 'We instructed our participants to do several acts of kindness each week for ten weeks,' she explains. Some were asked to mix their acts of kindness up, while others were requested to do the same thing at a similar time. 'The only ones who got happier were those who varied their generosities.'

The upshot seems to be that you alter your set point of happiness through *actual activities.* 'People often mistakenly think that you just "choose" to be happy,' says Dr Korb. 'But that's not how it works. You have to choose things that make you happy.' And the clincher is, he says, these things are frequently not *what we are told will make us happy.*

They're oftentimes ordinary drudgery, rather than extraordinary hedonism. They're things like meeting deadlines, going to the gym rather than swerving it, not eating junk and not spending your disposable income on designer trainers.

I have a list of '26 things that make me happy' (printed on page 41), most of which are free, and the rest of which cost under a tenner. Having them written down reminds me that when I engage in just a few of those activities every day, I'm happier. Simple.

Your activities will be entirely different to mine, but you already know what they are. Happiness is an activity.

SATISFICERS VS MAXIMIZERS

As if our negatively biased brains and the hedonic treadmill weren't enough to contend with, we also have a psychological phenomenon called 'maximizing'.

Some people are satisfied with their lot, and they tend to be called 'satisficers' by those in the know, whereas those who constantly reach are called 'maximizers'. A satisficer will spend maybe a few hours shopping for a new bed – a maximizer could spend days. A maximizer needs to eliminate every option and find the best one. A satisficer will clean the bits you can see when people come to stay. A maximizers will clean under things and scrub cupboards.

Take Steve Jobs. A classic maximizer. His wife Laurene was quoted saying that it took them *eight years* of discussion to decide upon a sofa. 'We spent a lot of time asking ourselves "What is the purpose of a sofa?"' she said. They were speedier when it came to choosing a washing machine. 'We spent about two weeks talking about this every night at the dinner table,' Jobs told *Wired* magazine.

Professor Paul Dolan sums this up nicely in his book *Happy Ever After: escaping the myth of the perfect life*. 'Maximizing involves searching until the very best option is identified by a process of elimination. The distinction was first put forward by Herbert Simon in the 1950s and has been popularized in recent times by Barry Schwarz,' he writes.

'A maximizer booking a holiday will spend hours – days even – sifting through the best deals online within budget,' continues Professor Dolan. 'They will weigh up all the options, taking account of all critical factors such as price, location, room size, breakfast offering, recent reviews and so on, and then will proudly announce "I have found the best possible deal". A satisficer will hit "Reserve" as soon as they come across the right sort of hotel within budget.'

Errrrr. Um. Given I have been known to spend upwards of six hours trawling websites for a holiday, I am without a doubt a maximizer. I suspect it's knitted into my DNA.

It's why, even though I don't judge my friends on the state of their skirting boards, I am fanatical about ensuring mine are dust-free when they come to stay.

It's why I don't shop for clothes frequently; instead I spend an entire day twice/three times a year going round all the shops and seeing *all the things*, before making choices. It's why I don't shop in metropolises, which are just too vast. I tend to go to much more manageable small cities or shopping centres; I can cover that ground; it's a 10k rather than a marathon.

As a maximizer on the hedonic treadmill, I tip that fecker up to the steepest incline. I want to be able to run 5km without stopping. Then 10km. Then to do a mini-triathlon. Then, then, then.

I have my sights set on a constantly shifting target. And who's moving it? I am. Nobody else *but me*.

How society encourages us to be maximizers

Society looks askance at satisficers and scratches its chin in confusion. Whereas maximizers get enabled by Mexican waves of affirmation.

I don't know many satisficers, but the couple I do know, are among the happiest people I've ever encountered. They choose to stay in their professions of hairdressing and building, rather than aspiring to own a hairdressers/be a foreman. They have chosen not to get married, not to have kids, and to rent rather than buy.

Society rewards them by constantly harassing them with questions as to what their career plans are, why they're not married, why they don't have kids, aren't they scared they'll regret not having them? They've told me they're really bored of responding 'We're happy as we are.' People don't know what the devil to make of them. So they try to pluck them from their satisfied sojourn, and to push them onto the treadmill too.

When I had just finished writing two books within eight months and was like a wrung rag, the most common question I was asked was, 'So, what's next? What's the next book?!'

Huh? Whoa there, Sparky. A rest. That's what's next.

It's the parent with the six-month-old who keeps being asked about having a second, the couple who've celebrated two years and are now batting back questions about engagement, or the person who's just bought a house who's being asked if they're going to extend it.

In the eyes of the madding crowd, being a satisficer means you're content with the fuzzy end of the lollipop. By being a maximizer and extra-seeking, you're not like those sad dipsticks who are settling for their awarded lot. You're trying to hoist yourself up by your britches, thanksabunch short-changing world.

Life for maximizers is a neverending escalator, not a lift where you – ping! –arrive at your desired floor. Your destination is a blinking, fizzing neon motel sign that seems to get further away, no matter how much of the desert you churn up, as if you're trapped in a trippy nightmare.

But, satisficers have it made. When I think of a satisficer, I think of this amazing quote from Simon Pegg. 'You could be living on a rock in the middle of the ocean, wearing a pair of Y-fronts, with a neverending supply of sandwiches. If that makes you happy, then you're a complete success, you know?'

WHEN I DIDN'T WANT TO
EXIST ANYMORE

'The extraordinary is not our homeland but the land of our
exile. The extraordinary is Babylon. It is the ordinary that is
our only homeland. How could we have been so deluded?'

Michael Foley, *Embracing the Ordinary*

I reached a place in 2013 where the pain of my existence outweighed the fear of
disappearing. I wanted to scratch myself out, as a person scratches off a golden
panel on a scratchcard.

My disillusion with life started to set in early. Very early.

Aged six, I remember sitting there, face sandwiched in my hands, staring
out of my Carrickfergus living room window for an entire day. Why? My
imaginative friend Judith had told me that she was sending a van full of My
Little Pony merchandise for me.

My face, which was initially lit up (like the Glo Worm I also coveted),
darkened as shadows started to fall. Eventually my mother asked what the
heck I was playing at. I told her, she chuckled, and called Judith a 'fantasist',
whatever that meant.

I trudged upstairs to my room, where I already had about 17 My Little
Ponys, and the castle, and the little dragon dude, and felt my first crushing
disappointment. It was the first time I can remember being truly dissatisfied
with my lot, and feeling I needed more.

The trend continued. In secondary school, we all idolized a girl called
Kimberley, because she had a pool in her garden, a perfect perm, a year-round
tan (second home in Spain), and every Benetton jumper it was possible to buy
at Merry Hill shopping centre. At my school, if you didn't have a Benetton
jumper you may as well have been dead. But my clothes mostly came from
Dudley market, which was far from a mecca of high fashion, and during PE, I
rocked Nick's trainers.

My decade of disenchantment

And so, I bolted into my twenties like a runaway horse, thinking that here was my chance to quell the have-not vibe of my teens.

But that too fell far short of my expectations. *Friends* has a lot to answer for, in my opinion, since I half expected that decade to be spent in a sexy turquoise-n-exposed brick loft, with a solid group of hilarious friends, playing ball games in the park, being able to afford endless coffee and muffins, as we supported each other through ladder-climbing and love-life-finessing.

I expected trials and tribulations. What I didn't expect was to live in rooms smaller than Carrie Bradshaw's walk-in wardrobe, in nine different rented flats across my twenties (*so much moving*).

One of the flats I lived in had rats that had clearly seen *Escape from Alcatraz*. They literally tunnelled their buck-toothed way into the fridge, by gnashing determinedly at a tiny defrosting hole, in order to plunder our ham and fruit. We thought it was each other doing the food-pinching. But after a few awkward, 'errr did you?' tip-toed chats, we established it wasn't. The true culprit was unmasked one night when we heard something crashing about in the utility room that turned out to furry, six-inches long and sporting a tail.

We asked the landlord, 'Can rats open fridge doors, because food is going missing?' at which he roared in laughter. But he soon backpedalled when he pulled the fridge out from the wall and discovered cheese cubes and melon lined up in a neat row, as if the ultimate picnic.

Then, I moved from the Midlands to London and expected a surfeit of intersectional friends as a cosmic reward, like when Laura Linney moved to Barbary Lane in *Tales of the City*.

Instead, I struggled to make friends in the mega-tropolis of faceless London, where it's illegal to look strangers in the eye.

I didn't expect my quest for the ultimate extraordinary night out to birth an alcohol addiction. If I was bored, I didn't go home. I drank more, in an attempt to salvage this faceplant of a night. Just one more drink, bar, dance. As a result of my shenanigans, I earned the nicknames 'Booze Hag' and 'Bad Santa'. (I have a picture of me in a Bad Santa hat someplace.)

I didn't expect to not be able to make a relationship last more than three years. I didn't anticipate having to do a Saturday job on top of my full-time job as an assistant on *Cosmopolitan* magazine, in order to pay astronomical London rent.

My friends were getting engaged, starting families even, and had gotten on the property ladder thanks to parents handing them deposits, or the bittersweet windfall of inheritance, and in comparison, I felt like the very definition of a loser. On my 27th birthday, my mates made me a birthday book which they all wrote and drew in; all of the doodles of me starred wine and cigarettes. Later that night, I would chip my front tooth by drunkenly falling into a front door.

My disappointment in myself manifested itself in my criticism of everything around me. I was hard on myself, and thus hard on the rest of my world. If a friend commented, 'this coffee is lovely', I'd cast my mind back to the coffee I'd had that was better. A boyfriend would take me for a picnic in Kew Gardens for my birthday, and I moaned to my mates later that he didn't pack any wine. I needed a cuff around the ear.

Losing an imaginary race

And thus I spent my twenties perpetually disappointed, panicking and pissed off. I entered my early thirties in a blind panic at the life boxes I still hadn't managed to tick. I couldn't even see the boxes, let alone climb inside to tick them.

I thought by the end of my twenties I'd have a ring on it and a mortgage for a flat with window boxes; possibly a baby blooming in my belly too. That didn't happen. (That *still* hasn't happened.) I felt visceral shame for failing to achieve the golden triad of Spouse! House! Babies!

By 30, I had the job I'd wanted, as a Features Editor on a million-selling newspaper supplement, but I hated every hothoused second of it, and in under a year I'd failed and bailed, and had to move back home for six months as a result of a total lack of savings.

I felt like everyone was ahead of me, even though they weren't. That no matter how hard I ran, I didn't feel satisfied long-term, beyond a brief vault of triumph about the promotion, or the moving-in, or the whatever. That vault was always short-lived; a long jump that wound up in my eating sand. Followed by flatlining and feeling the same as I had done before the realization of vaultin' ambition.

At the grand age of 32, I spent my birthday gulpy-sobbing because I'd just been dumped and I felt 'old' (seems laughable now, but I truly felt like that) and like 'time was running out' and that 'I was going to end up alone'.

The guy I was seeing wasn't even a big love, he was just another dude with whom I cried The One, in order to attempt to solve the problem of my singleness. I felt as if I was trapped inside a giant egg timer, and sand was being sucked from beneath my feet.

I didn't even know what the hedonic treadmill was, or that it existed inside my head, and yet I still felt haunted by that unnamed urge. I started getting so tired of dating, of pitching ideas, of just about hustling together my rent, of trying and failing to save. The idea of saving £40K – the 20 per cent deposit needed for an average flat in London at the time – seemed utterly preposterous, so why bother even saving £400?

I was increasingly opting to slide off the treadmill and sit beside it instead, smoking and sinking wine in order to anaesthetize my despair, which was blossoming like a bruise.

As a result, my peers got further and further ahead, and I felt more and more hopeless each time I contemplated where I was, and how fast I would have to skedaddle in order to catch up. I had hedonic treadmill ennui, but no name for it.

I didn't know back then, that many of my friends were extraordinary, and that I was actually very ordinary. I didn't know that most people *didn't* get married in their late twenties or early thirties; I didn't know that most of my peers were renting too.

I just-so-happened to make friends with over-achievers. And I chose to focus all my energy on chasing them, rather than regarding those running alongside me.

Something inside me starts to tick

Suicidal ideation has been represented as sinking into uncharted depths, being shadowed by a black dog, or falling into the empty spaces between words.

For me, it was more like unwittingly building a bomb. Its motherboard? Extraordinary expectations.

Over the years, I accidentally collected more and more bomb-assembly parts. (Drinks far too much, check. Attracted to men who aren't that bothered about me, check. Allows money to burn a hole in pocket, check. Alienates work contacts, check.)

Once I had enough parts, the device just fell together of its own accord, like a bunch of magnets, and started to tick.

I'd even mentally written the note I would BluTack to the door to stop my cohabiting boyfriend from coming in and finding me. 'I'm sorry, I can't live in my own skin anymore. Please don't come into this room. Please call an ambulance instead.'

And one night, I got into a bathtub with a kitchen knife at 3am, inconsolable, and willed myself to do something. I lay there for an hour, until the water was goosebump cold. For that hour, I existed in between two worlds; not wanting to live, yet not being able to do what was necessary to die.

In retrospect, that night was a dress rehearsal. I hadn't stuck the note to the door, so I now know that my suicidal ideation was just that. An idea. My device was still ticking, and had not yet reached the final countdown.

I think I was doing a trial run, to see if I could use the knife, and I couldn't. Turns out that even though I wanted to cease existing, I was still a wuss when it came to pain.

The next day I started Googling 'Painless ways to commit suicide', hoping to hit upon an answer that wouldn't involve blood, agony or seizures. Instead of finding a 'how to', I found a deterrent site, masquerading as a how to.

It jolted me awake by telling me – via capitals, the grammatical version of shouting – that 'THERE IS NO PAINLESS WAY' and 'YOU WILL CAUSE YOUR LOVED ONES GREAT DISTRESS IF YOU MANAGE IT'. It was like a punch in the nose.

But to be honest, the follow-up, 'Also, you'll probably fail and live the rest of your life in agony, a burden to family who will then have to feed you and wipe your bottom' was more of a deterrent.

I believed my loved ones despised me anyhow, despite much evidence to the contrary, so the only hopeful future I could envisage was that of them throwing me a sensational funeral, probably with a soundtrack featuring Jeff Buckley and Fleetwood Mac, and then going back to their new-and-improved lives, minus me.

But, my ideation never materialized into action, because what I wanted was an absence of pain. To press a button and make myself – whoosh! – vanish. I didn't want *more* pain before non-existence. Or the prospect of potential failure ('I can't even get suicide right'), paralysis and my carers (which would undoubtedly be my family) then loathing me even more than they did already (or so I thought).

So, that website probably saved my life. The next day I called my father and asked for help. I'd assessed all pain options – suicide, continuing to drink and be depressed, or quitting drinking and finding a way out of depression – and decided that changing was the best option.

Tony Robbins isn't normally my guru of choice, but he hit the nail precisely on the head when he said, 'Change happens when the pain of staying the same is greater than the pain of change'.

I set about dismantling the bomb inside me, trying to tick me to my untimely demise.

'Life is so constructed that the event does not, cannot, will not, match the expectation.'

Charlotte Brontë

I LOCATE THE EXACTITUDE
OF GRATITUDE

The reasons I got into that bathtub with that knife were threefold. I had been kidnapped by addiction; both love and booze, with which I was in Stockholm Syndrome enmeshment. But also, I had a 'poor me' (pour me another) mentality. I was stuck in a victim storyline.

I had typecast myself as the put-upon. I couldn't come to terms with my ordinary looks, my stalling career, my common-or-garden existence as a thirtysomething renter, my financial existence on the precipice of my overdraft, or my ordinary body.

I was in a constantly reaching state. Better – more – faster – where's mine? What I totally failed to realize was that my future happiness was not on a shelf slightly out of my reach. It was already all around me, buried in the ordinary experiences I was having on a day-to-day basis, the experiences I saw as wasted time until I upgraded; the holding bay of life until I entered the real deal by getting everything I thought I wanted.

So, how did I go from disappointed kid, through disenchanted wanker, into utterly despondent, and then born-again enchanted? (I saw that eye roll.)

I saw a post in a Facebook group for the newly sober, which was a shout-out for assembling a Gratitude Group, based on the hunch that 'a grateful heart never drinks'.

I simultaneously pulled towards it, while my Britishness tried to pull me away. But I was desperate enough to contain my 'corny!' knee-jerk, and try it anyhow.

Why gratitude literature is offputting

Most articles about gratitude leave me cold, despite gratitude itself being smackyouawake powerful. They make me feel like I ought to be cross-stitching 'Thank you Lord' onto a cushion. Or chanting 'I am not worthy of this offering' before a bread basket.

Here are some real lines from real gratitude literature, plus how I felt when I read them. (Article origins and writers obviously concealed.)

- **Don't be picky. Appreciate everything.**

Hmm, really? Everything? Next they'll be telling me to do some 'mindful washing up'; enjoying the warm water on my hands, and the slide of soap over my fingers, oh lucky me.

No thanks. My gratitude is not about appreciating *everything*, because that's disingenuous.

- **You may not like your job, but at least you have a job.**

This is true, but man, does the tone annoy me.

OK, so the likelihood is that if you can afford to buy this book, you had an education, and live someplace where your family aren't likely to get killed by machine-gun-brandishing guerrillas, and you have a dwelling with four walls and a roof, and don't have to steal food in order to eat. This is all undeniably true.

But because we're surrounded by others who are in the same fortunate position, it's very easy to slide into the mentality of alighting on first world problems. I know. I've done it. *I do it.*

It's all very 'Overheard in Waitrose/Whole Foods' and is the mentality of 'my tenth pair of shoes are too tight, my new iPhone is too big, my warm flat is too small, the sunrise is too bright'.

It's human, it's natural, and we all do it, not because we're spoilt brats, but because of hedonic adaptation.

Scolding 'check your privilege!' articles like this are very much in the 'there are starving children in...' vein. Yes, there are, and we damn straight shouldn't forget it, and we should stay aware and donate money/help if we can, but that does not mean that people in the first world are disallowed from having negative feelings.

Being fortunate in the grand scheme, and yet unhappy, are two things that often co-exist. Are *allowed* to co-exist.

- **Practising gratitude means paying attention to what we are grateful for.**

No shit, Sherlock. But how? HOW? This is way too vague. Bah.

Creating micro, rather than macro gratitude

So, let's dig into the 'how'. Gratitude is an activity that you need to engage in. I know so many people who claim to 'do' gratitude, but actually do nothing.

They think it's just a vague feeling of thankfulness. But you have to *do it*, in order to *get it*. Claiming to be a practitioner of gratitude without doing anything is like reading about running, rather than getting out there and experiencing the brain-rush of endorphins for real. Or claiming you can fly a plane, when all you can do is operate a Playstation flight simulator.

It's really easy to blahdiblah about an 'attitude of gratitude', but here I want to talk about an 'exactitude of gratitude'. Locating and lassoing the exact moments in the workaday that are lovely.

Many people who try to do gratitudes go too big. They write lists that say things like:

I'm grateful for my job.

I'm grateful for my dog.

I'm grateful for food in the fridge.

And they find that they then tend to write the same things over and over, because they have the same dog, and job, and fridge food, and therefore the gratitude listing has no power. It just becomes like a mirror mantra we recite and yet don't believe. It's saying 'I am enough' rather than drilling down to why you think you're not enough. To get to the core of gratitude, it's all about sourcing the specific.

Indeed, a 2005 psychological study found that when we re-play the same gratitudes over and over, they start to have way less impact. It's like when you set a song that makes you happy as your alarm clock tune. Over time, the re-play of the song begins to produce indifference, rather than heart-soaring joy.

Then, the song no longer makes you happy, it actually irritates you.* Re-played gratitudes lose their joy too.

This rule of the diminishing returns of repetition is why robotically listing your standard grocery-list blessings *does not work*. What does work is finding new beauties that are unique to the day.

I didn't know any of this back when I started writing nightly gratitude lists. However, one of the golden rules of magazine and newspaper writing is to 'make it as specific as possible', rather than using sweeping statements, and so I

---

* Eventually, it makes you murderous. And lo and behold, you have ruined one of your favourite songs through repetition.

was used to homing in on specifics. I'd just been trained to do so.

I remember one of my bosses telling me that if an interviewee was talking about finding their husband dead in the kitchen, you had to deny your humanity and get past the horror of that revelation, and to delve awkwardly into the specifics. That after expressing empathy, the key questions to ask were: what colour were the kitchen tiles? Was there the smell of anything cooking? Can you remember what *exactly* you were wearing...oh and what day of the week was it?

So, entirely by accident, I alit upon a gratitude practice that was micro, rather than macro. And thus I blundered upon a goldmine, because if your gratitudes are specific sights, or feelings, or conversations, or things from that particular day, it means they're never *Groundhog Day* repetitive, and thus the power of them, in my experience, doesn't wear off.

Micro gratitudes I've written

- Today I lay reading on the sofa wearing just my pants, listening to Alabama Shakes and drinking fresh mint tea that was like a garden party in my mouth. Was nice.

- Nobody told me adult life would involve so much cardboard. But today I decided to see it as destruction therapy, like when people pay to go and smash things up in 'rage rooms' (real thing). I razed through it with a scalpel, leapt on it in boots and got the playhouse proportioned stash of 'just in case' bubble wrap and jumped on that too. So satisfying.

- When I was growing up, a '3D cinema' involved going to a weird theatre with moving chairs, where you had water squirted at you and stale air blown up your bum. It was odd. Today, we paid just over a tenner and felt like we were soaring over mountains on the back of a dragon.

- I just pressed a few buttons on an app, rather than had a painful five-minute phonecall, and a nice person on a moped brought me a bag of food devised in another continent to my door. If I had a person from the 1950s with me right now, they'd be like, 'What is this actual sorcery?'

- Today's walk, which featured a murder of crows on a watchtower wire, set against a slash of neon yellow, as if the field on the horizon had been highlighted for being particularly inspirational. Then a sheepdog splushed towards us through the long grass, with a pink hair slide in her silver hair keeping her eyes free to see.

- That I felt that camera flash of pain in my gob that tells me I need to go to the dentist – so I went to the dentist. That I can now afford to do so, without financial jiggery-pokery and stress.

- There are a pair of swallows raising a family outside my kitchen window that I have finally gotten to trust me, through time and persistence. At first they would wheel away, chirping madly when I came to the window. Now, they sit there, serene, looking me straight in the eyes. Getting a bird to trust you is a rush.

- That I chose to swerve bubblegum for the brain this evening in the shape of a Rebel Wilson film, and watched the nourishing Netflix documentary *Given*, which made me re-frame swimming as flying underwater.

- For a night-time run in driving diagonal wind, the type that slows your progress almost to a halt, or makes you feel like you may take flight. The kind of hungry waves that make you wonder how the pier hasn't been relocated underwater, like some sort of Atlantis featuring a funfair. And makes you marvel how the wind farm on the horizon, blinking red like an oncoming robot army, is still upright.

- For the reminder from Instagrammer Florence Given that 'Women don't owe you pretty'. Today I gave myself permission to be ~~ugly~~ make-up free in the sweet country air.

- Today a very macho male friend told me that, sometimes, he pretends he's stretching against a tree and when nobody's looking, he gives it a quick cuddle. It makes me snort every time I think of it.

- Today my friend Holly and I played the fun 'what do you see in this abstract art' game and I basically saw things a seven-year-old would see ('I see an owl delivering post') while she saw religious iconography ('I see the Virgin Mary').

- Today my five-year-old niece zeroed in on my tampon like a sniper. 'What's that?' she enquired, her antennae for adult things twitching.
I answered.
'What's a period?'
I explained.
And then, after a beat of a pause, she said:
'What's a *pagina*?'

- For this gorgeous lyric by Van Morrison in *Astral Weeks* – 'If I ventured in the slipstream between the viaducts of your dreams'.

- Today I bought myself a mini packet of Ferrero Rocher rather than whingeing about other people never buying me the nutty planets of joy; now I feel like I have gained mastery over my own chocolate galaxy.*

- Washing my hands in a coffee shop bathroom, I looked up expecting to see a mirror, and instead saw an empty frame with, 'You're beautiful, just as you are' in it.

The science of gratitude

It's well peddled that we have a genetically pre-determined set point for happiness, which stays more or less the same (unless something wildly horrific happens, such as the death of a child). What isn't as widely known is that some experts think that only 50 per cent of our happiness is pre-determined, while 10 per cent is circumstance, and the remaining 40 per cent is influenced by what we do ('intentional activity').

And one of the ways we can change that malleable 40 per cent is undoubtedly: gratitudes. There are hundreds, maybe even thousands of studies that back this up.

I tend to write my gratitudes just before bed. If I don't, whether because I'm travelling or ~~having sex~~ have company, I find that my mind takes longer to stop swirling enough to fall asleep.

If you're going to get stuck into gratitude listing too, writing too many can actually backfire, says Professor Lyubomirsky. 'We're doing a study right now in which we've asked participants to list two, four, eight, 16 or 32 blessings (or

---

* This gratitude was not sponsored by Ferrero Rocher.

things they're grateful for) per day. Our results are showing that eight is the most effective number.'

Neuroscientist Dr Korb adds that it's best to keep each gratitude snappy, rather than going into too much depth (note to self to keep them shorter). 'Writing, analysing and using language activates the prefrontal cortex, which is great for reducing the intensity of negative memories, but on the flipside, it can also reduce the intensity of positive memories,' he explains.

'So rather than writing at length about what exactly happened, keep it brief,' suggests Dr Korb. The objective is to summon, rather than scrutinize. 'You want to visualize, but not analyse; analysing will suck the enjoyment out of the memory's recall.' Writing in depth about a trauma is a great idea, but with gratitude-ing, short is the sweet spot.

Outward-facing gratitude

Directing gratitude outward, rather than keeping it locked in your lists, also has a profound effect. A University of Pennsylvania study unearthed the finding that sending a 'thank you' letter delivered a happiness boost to the sender that lasted *a whole month.*

'Some research shows that gratitude letters can be even more powerful than lists,' says Professor Lyubomirsky. 'Even if you don't send them to the people they're about, the letters are often complex, detailed and rich.'

I used to send the gratitudes that mentioned specific people to the actual person, because I wanted them to feel my gratitude, rather than leaving it trapped in my computer. But I only did this for the first year or so, as it became unsustainable, and everyone started thinking I was an oddball. ('John, Cath keeps texting me about how grateful she is for me...do you think she's losing it?')

I also now direct gratitudes to myself, for whenever I go swimming, or do dull admin, or cook from scratch when I really don't feel like it. When you demonstrate gratitude towards someone, they're more likely to perform that action more often. And that *someone* includes yourself.

If writing isn't your *thing*, then there's no apparent reason why other forms of 'gratitude listing' would not have the same well-being whack. Visualizing exactly what happened in order to relive it; keeping a daily gratitude photo diary; drawing doodles; or, if you're more of a talker than a scribe, recording your gratitudes via voice note.

A silver marker pen for the awful

Some things are devastating, and I'm not going to take that away from you, or ask you to deny the unavoidable negatives of life.

The death of a loved one, a miscarriage, a serious illness; you are allowed to be sideswiped and floored by these things, rather than goaded into seeing the silver linings of every cloud, or somesuch insulting pat.

However, if you go one floor down to the 'also truly awful, but not quite as awful' level of job losses, infidelities or having to move house, these appear to have no trace of good about them, at first glance. But I've experienced all of them in the past six years, and have realized that if I can't find even a sliver of a silver lining, I now have a fat marker pen with which to draw it in myself.

Say a relationship ends; now I know he's a cheater. Or if a boring but reliable source of income vanishes; now I can pursue something that doesn't turn my brain into a narcoleptic. Having to move house; a new town becomes my oyster.

At first glance, it seems insulting, even reductive to the undeniable smackdown of these experiences, but it's ultimately a favour to ourselves. Given we can't change the thing, we may as well try to trace a positive outline around the thing, right?

Essentially, what I've learned from my gratitude experiment is this: the extraordinary is not where the cellular-level happiness is at. It's in the ordinary.

Infinitesimal workaday moments that are a brief flash of sunlight. An almond croissant, an inquisitive robin hopping around you, finding a fiver you'd forgotten about, shopping delivered to your door*. Once we re-frame things that we take for granted, things that we're like 'oh, that's just *there*', we can see it through fresh eyes.

Or, once you focus on the alleviation of a hard thing, rather than the hard thing, this shift can transmute your grouchy mood into grateful. Cue:

- The snap of shutting your laptop after a late night and entering the navy velvet liberty of the evening, rather than counting how many extra minutes unpaid overtime you had to do.

- Instead of focusing on the sloshy walk home from the train station in hammering rain, registering the lovely swish-clunk-dunk of double locking

---

* Mentally time-travel to tell your 2001 self about this. Look at how chuffed they are.

your front door, peeling off your wet clothes, enjoying the bloom of a hot shower on a cold body, and knowing you don't have to go out again.

- The pleasure of finally eating after a long wait, rather than concentrating on the length of the wait.

Just as a photographer finds a focal point in a picture, and gets it pin-sharp, blurring the rest of the scene, that's what we can do too. Fuzz the bad; sharpen the good.

Gratitude is just a way of adding to your invincible summer, a mental utopia all of us have the power to create. 'The existentialist Albert Camus wrote about an "invincible summer" that exists in all of us – deep positive memories that can carry us through difficult times,' says Dr Korb.

Perception is a powerful thing. We can alter ours voluntarily. Physically *changing our brain* from a bad-seeking missile, into a good-finding lighthouse. And the person who will benefit the most from that? Ourselves. Gratitude lists might seem like the psychological equivalent of wearing an excruciatingly twee 'Begin each day with a grateful heart' T-shirt, but they're actually counter-culture, self-serving, radical neuroplasticity.

'The research participants who had the ability to lean fully into joy only shared one variable in common...gratitude. They practised gratitude...I get so busy sometimes chasing the extraordinary moments that I don't pay attention to the ordinary moments. The moments that if taken away, I would miss more than anything.'

Brené Brown, *The Call to Courage*, Netflix

26 THINGS THAT MAKE ME HAPPY

As we now know, happiness is an activity, and these everyday things spark joy for me.

1.   Prowling the park for cute dogs to pet, and saying 'Can I?' to bemused owners.
2.   Having secret races with people on the seafront/in the park. Given they don't know, I frequently win.
3.   Learning to fix things myself via the magical learning portal of YouTube.
4.   Buying a fridgeful of food and dropping off a tenner's worth to a food bank on the way home.
5.   Talking to my plants. Feel free to call me a nutcase, but ever since I've been like 'Hello beautiful, damn, you look *fine* today', I haven't had one plant die on me. My plants are clearly narcissists.
6.   Keeping on top of my emails. Exceptionally boring, but true.
7.   Helping someone who is prodding futilely at a ticket machine, can't use the office coffee machine, or is struggling with a pram on steps. There's a cruel big-city irony that we're less likely to help each other as our numbers increase. Let's make a big-city pact, right now. Are you in?
8.   Make-up off, hair washed, PJs on at 8pm. Rock and indeed roll.
9.   Paying bills before they're due, and feeling like a fiscal mastermind.
10. Being touched, and no, not necessarily like that. Holding a friend's hand, someone stroking my inner forearm, a cuddle from a cat; these all count.
11. Remembering people's birthdays.
12. Catching a spider and releasing it back into the wild. Remembering I am thousands of times larger than it, and that *Arachnophobia* was a work of fiction.
13. Running boldly into the icy sea, only to run right back out. But still, boy, does that make me feel alive.
14. Browsing online galleries of tiny homes, houseboats and tree houses. Seeing how other people live joyfully with so little space.

15. Going on an obsessive deep-dive once I discover a new artist, writer or thinker.

16. A game of basketball, tennis or ping pong. Anything with balls, basically. Balls make me happy. Yes, you can quote me on that.

17. Giving a stranger a compliment a day, whether it's that their front garden is gorgeous, their hat is rad, or their rainbow hair is the coolest hair I've ever seen.

18. Stapling things. Sometimes I staple things that really do not require stapling, just because the ker-chung makes me feel efficient. Dream gift: a staple gun.

19. Going to a pier/arcade and spending a few quid on whack-a-mole, 2p machines and car-racing games.

20. Writing. Anything. Even shopping lists. It makes my brain feel unpacked.

21. Deep-sea nature programmes. I love looking out onto the silvery Atlantic and knowing that someplace in that body of water, there are whales gliding around like aquatic Zeppelins and seahorses that look like seven-inch dragons.

22. Kitchen dancing. Anarchistic moods bring out hair-tossing to Hole or Cypress Hill, or if I'm euphoric it's Simple Minds or Phoenix. My kitchen sees a lot of questionable moves.

23. Using words that sound like what they're describing. Roundabout. Mist. Helter-skelter. Sneaky. Sparkle.

24. Treating rush-hour pavements as if they're an obstacle course I need to zip through as deftly as possible. It turns a thousand-person-strong hellscape into an agility test.

25. On a cold day, turning the heating on and getting back into bed with a coffee.

26. Hanging with the people I love, and meeting new ones. Even though my introverted streak always tries to talk me out of going to the gathering, I never regret *having gone*.

II: ORDINARY LIVING

ODES TO THE ORDINARY
An ode to not emigrating

'I'm so bored of living here!' say people in Sicily, New Zealand, Ireland, Canada, Norway, the Gold Coast, California…It's part of the human condition to *want to live where you don't live*. We hedonically adapt to where we live to such an extent that we no longer see its beauty.

A Gallup world poll discovered that the desire to emigrate grew dramatically between 2015 and 2017, with 15 per cent of adults worldwide now wanting to bugger off and live someplace else.

In the same way that people have a Band-Aid baby to attempt to fix a wounded relationship, many emigrate under the misconception it will mend their lives. 'Yet wherever you go, there you are', smugs the bumper sticker.

We live in a society that now derides those who stay still as unimaginative backwater buzzkills, and awards brave, outward-facing, cosmopolitan-AF trophies to those who move around.

Those who move are definitely brave, but sometimes, and I speak from personal experience here, their many moves are propelled by a jetpack of mistakes. Frequent movers can often be fleeing relationships and situations that have gotten messy. Where are the awards for those who stay still? Who ride out skirmishes in small towns, or patch up frayed relationships, or reinvent inherited homes?

I've always had gypsy blood. And a hankering to live someplace extraordinary, someplace abroad, which is why I've previously lived in both Bruges and Barcelona (only the Bs apparently) for around the same (or less) than it would cost to rent a place in London. I've always sneered at those who stay still.

And yet, what these geolocation-swapping experiments turned up was: I prefer home. The million cutesy 'There's no place like home, y'all' tin-and-rope kitchen signs could well be right. Just like with a romantic partner, often you don't know what you've got until it's gone.

Around Bruges, the geometrically perfect lines of the countryside, the spirit-level straight horizon, the trees and bushes 'scaped within an inch of their lives, meant that when I returned to my homeland, I was beside myself over the curves and imperfectness of our green and pleasant land. And the soil! I didn't fully appreciate our bouncy soil until trying to run on the packed, arid soil of Spain.

Wherever your home is, sometimes you need to interrupt the experience of it in order to appreciate it anew (remember, from page 21 about how interrupting pleasure intensifies it?). It's why you might come back from the lush, sexy greenery of Cambodia and sigh deeply at being greeted by the Mars-scape plains of Vegas. It's why sweet, low-lying suburbia can grow suffocating, but then be resuscitated by a spell of having been leaned upon by shard-like skyscrapers. It's why Australians move to Europe, and then mostly back again; and vice versa.

Similarly, we always want what we haven't got when it comes to weather. But once we get what we don't have, we re-think it. Our skin capabilities, disposition and preference are almost always auto-tuned to the place we're originally from. Irish people generally can't abide African heat, there is no SPF high enough. Meanwhile, Bajans think even a sunny day in Brussels is bloody freezing. It's why on holiday, the locals 'brrrr!' in full shirts and trousers while I sit in a bikini with sweat inelegantly dripping off my nose.

I thought I was going to love living someplace with perpetually sunny weather. Show me the sun and I will lie in it, along with the mad dogs. You have to drag me out of a sauna. However, it actually became mundane that the Barcelonian weather was a steady sunshiny minimum of 30 degrees (*hedonic adaptation*, yo).

Instead, I grew to love the breaks in the monotony; the showboating, monthly Catalan thunderstorms during which I thought the sky was going to crack in two, and I suddenly understood why my local friend said, 'people stay home when it rains here' given the streams flowing down the streets, stealing tourist's flip flops.

When you're hot all the time, you miss being cold. It's why, in balmy countries, they're fixated on air-conditioning shops until your teeth chatter. There is something so luxurious about lowering yourself into a bath when you're chilled to the blood; it feels like a full-body orgasm. Not to mention the bliss of taking a hot-water bottle to bed and curling around it.

Also, when a sunny day arrives, it's in my British bone marrow to sprint to the nearest park, skedaddle to the beach, or more accurately, sit in long traffic jams to the nearest park or beach. Brits are trained to make the most of it.

What I found is this: the sun-salute guilt never leaves you. Even into my third month of Barcelona, I felt a smudge of guilt about being inside working or cleaning or just hanging on a sunny day, which was practically every day. So, there's that.

Sunbathing is something you only really have proper time to do when on holiday. When you live someplace exotic, you are only year-round tanned if you really commit to the cause. Around a month in, I was walnut brown, but by the end of my three-month stay, I was almost back to normal. Because sunbathing is best reserved for small doses on holiday.

You need to put the hours in; you're not just auto-tanned because you now live in Spain. The melanin Gods do not auto-tan you because they can see that you now pay your rent to a Barcelonian.

I'm not saying I didn't enjoy the sunshine there, of course I did, but I am saying that it has given me the opposite of what I thought it would: a new-found appreciation for our up-and-down middlin' climate. I love a rainy Saturday now, as it is carte blanche to just rest and chill. I no longer hanker to permanently reside where it's predominately hot and sunny.

But most of all, I missed people speaking the same language as me. At first, I loved that I didn't understand the conversations of those around me, it was like white noise. I obviously learnt some basic phrases to get by, but having an actual conversation was beyond me, so unless they spoke great English, my daily communications were limited to scintillating exchanges such as, 'How much is this?', 'Table for two please', 'Yes I would like a receipt'.

I also missed the constant apologizing that goes on in Britain. Sorry you just bumped into me, terribly sorry 'bout that. Sorry I am standing in a place where you would also like to be! Sorry, but can I just ask you to do the job I am paying you to do? Sorry I'm alive! It's a curious national treasure, this apology always falling from our lips.

What we take utterly for granted as 'ordinary', is actually 'extraordinary' to those visiting our homes. I remember an Australian friend stopping in her tracks at the sight of a squirrel and insisting we sit and watch him crunch through a monkey nut for 20 minutes (and take 20 pictures of him), just as I would sit and be spellbound by a koala bear kipping on a branch.

While running alongside a beach in Palma, I stopped dead at what was, for me, an extraordinary sight. A cat, swirled on a beach rock, licking its paw. Hell's bells. I had never seen a cat on a beach before. I hunched down to take a picture of this anomaly, and wondered why no one else was doing the same. Then I ran on and saw dozens of cats. Yeah. It's a thing there.

While abroad, I've exclaimed with delight over the black-on-pink polka dots of dragon fruit – 'it's like the fruit version of an eighties party dress!' – and have then realized that since apples are $10 for four out there, Thai people probably feel the same way when they're given Pink Lady apples.

Now I remember. One person's squirrel is another's beach cat. And those who stay put – living someplace they were born maybe, or just choosing a town and growing roots – should be just as congratulated as those who whirl around like dervishes.

Stillness is equally as challenging, if not more so, than movement.

WHY EXTRA STUFF MEANS EXTRA 'SHOULDS'

I'm standing in the street, looking into a van, close to tears.

'Man, this is hard,' I say to the bewildered van driver. He shuffles side-to-side awkwardly.

He tries to shut the door.

'I just want one last look,' I plead, prising the door back open.

No, I wasn't parting ways with a beloved pet, or person, or even beloved *things*. I was giving away half of my stuff; stuff I quite simply never use/read/wear. And yet, it was a wrench.

Last night, before the van came I woke up in the middle of the night and urgently fished out a skirt from one of the bin bags; a skirt that no longer fits. It sits in my wardrobe, a symbol of my inability to completely let go.

It's not like I haven't edited this shit. I've moved house about, Christ knows, 12 times since leaving university. No, I'm not a fugitive (that I know of), but I did a) Rent, which meant if the owners chose to sell, I was out on my ear b) Move in with boyfriends I barely knew c) Drink myself blotto until age 33, so climates with housemates tended to frost over after a year or so.

When I moved house last year, I managed to fill a moving van the size of a shipping container. So, unless I wanted to require a fleet of HGVs for my next move, it became abundantly clear that I needed to purge. I needed to downgrade from my 'extra' amount of stuff.

We fill the space we're in

Have you moved house lately? And had that epiphany of 'Holy smokes, how do I have so much stuff'? Much like water pouring into an underground cave, or like air pushing its way into the corners of an inflatable mattress, we tend to expand to fill whatever space we're in.

I used to be able to fit my stuff into a teeny tiny room in a shared house, plus a separate wardrobe (there was literally no room for a wardrobe in my room) and a coupla boxes in the garage. Now, my stuff fills an entire flat made of four rooms, which is fivefold the size of the previous square footage I occupied.

And, we're not the only species with a predisposition to hoard. Squirrels tuck away treasure troves of nuts in hollow trees, hence our use of 'squirrel' away. Crocodiles create grisly underwater 'pantries' of kills. Magpies are suckers for jewellery, coins and trinkets, while black kites have evolved a sign o' the times predilection for using white plastic to decorate their nests. 'Octopus's Garden' is not just a Beatles song, it's a seabed fact, with the creatures assembling shiny things and shells, much as Aunt Maud collects garden-centre cherub statues.

Acquiring is fun. Possessing, less so.

The ancestry of stuff-hoarding is something Professor Cregan-Reid has been fascinated by. 'Storage only became necessary when we started acquiring more than we needed,' explains the author of *Primate Change*. 'First, Homo Sapiens invented jars, then shelves, then cupboards. Fast-forward a few thousand years and we now need the fluorescent storage metropolises that skirt our towns and cities. These are places where we dump our things because we no longer have space for them, because the pleasure of acquisition is greater than that of possession.'

Therein lies an extremely salient point. *The pleasure of acquisition is greater than that of possession.* Look at the clothes in your wardrobe. D'you remember the day you bought them? The day you put that jumpsuit – or that shirt – on in a changing room and thought 'this is going to change my life'.

Is it just me that thinks clothes have that level of cosmic significance sewn into them? And then you get it home and, ever so gradually, the sorcery you felt in the shop ebbs away. Yet, it's the same garment. It hasn't changed. Only your perception of it has. Your brain chemistry has changed in response to it.

And yet, says Professor Cregan-Reid, we're not hardwired to collect stuff. It's nurture, not nature. 'In evolutionary terms, having stuff would have been hugely disadvantageous. We migrated and moved with climate change; there were no caravans back then to take things with us. It wasn't until the Agricultural Revolution 10,000 years ago that we stopped moving. Which seems a really long time ago, but given Homo Sapiens have been around for two million years, it's a mere eyeblink.'

Our paranoia – clutching of – our possessions has evolved. In hunter-gatherer groups, kids were allowed to play with precious belongings such as knives. 'Any damage done was a valuable rite of passage. They needed to know about knives,' says Cregan-Reid. 'But once we started settling and farming, the lesson changed; kids were nurtured into protecting possessions at all costs. And being very careful with them. If a kid leaves a gate open and lets a herd of sheep out, that's a huge loss. The more stuff you have, the more you have to lose.'

Make do and...whack it on the credit card

Baby Boomers were the first generation that really could hoard, given they grew up in the first wave of the mass-produced, imported, 'Made in China', cheap-as-chips stuff tsunami. They merrily shoved the 'Make do and Mend' cross-stitch of the WWII generation into the back of a cupboard, and blockaded it with all of their buy-one-get-one-free scores. They were also the first generation to grow up in the age of credit cards; globally, the first one launched in 1950, while the first British credit card arrived in 1966.

This is why, oftentimes, when you walk into a Baby Boomer's house, you get the sensation that were their house to sneeze, drawers would shoot out, cupboards would fly open and stuff would wheeee! through the air, like in an enchanted Disney castle.

Generation X-ers and Millennials supposedly know better, given we trot out that much-peddled psyche truism, 'experiences make us happier than stuff' and constantly ask each other if we've 'seen that Netflix documentary on the Minimalists?'

But we learnt this propensity to 'just in case' hoard from Baby Boomers, which is why there is such a mania for de-cluttering, now that we know the stuff isn't the square root of all happiness. You can't de-clutter without clutter, so clearly we are just as hoardsome.

When the shoulds drove away

So, about three years after everyone else*, I watched some of that Marie Kondo TV show, and Kon-Maried the shit out of my flat. 'Does this tea towel spark joy?'

I assembled so much that my local charity shop sent that van to pick it up. And after my initial resistance, offloading it felt spec-freaking-tacular. Because, as soon as it drove off, all of these things drove away too.

'I should wear that.'

'I should use this present I don't want.'

---

* I like to be late on trends, given my 'not doing that if everyone else is' vibe makes me feel somewhat subversive *flicks imaginary cigarette and snarls*.

'I should read that.'

'I should be the kind of person who makes bread with this.'

'I should mend this thing I broke in 2009 and have been carting around ever since.'

Those shoulds are heavy. So much more heavy than the stuff.

The purge has also made me re-think books. Marie Kondo doesn't house more than 30 books, at any one time. Um, I practically had that *beside my bed*, in a wobbly tower. A tower that glowered at me. Even my bedside table was an astronomically unachievable to-do list.

'You just spent three hours watching Netflix,' the books would say. 'Rather than enriching your brain with us.'

'Why haven't you read me yet?' another whispered. 'You bought me over a year ago. Lazy cow.'

Now I have dismantled the glowering guilt tower and only keep one book beside my bed (at most two, if that book is too dense and I need something lighter as a foil). The rest hide away in a holding bay, so that I can't see them. Feels better. Much better.

Yes, Elon Musk may have read two books a day during his teens (says his brother), but why am I comparing myself to a stone cold genius?! Apparently, 51 per cent of British adults didn't read a book in 2018. So, I am winning, and so are you probably, simply by virtue of reading *this* book. And yet I constantly beat myself up for not reading enough, even though – given I get through dozens of books a year – I would be categorized as a 'heavy' reader by British standards.

Here's what I've learned. Humans are happier in an ordinary amount of stuff, rather than assembling a pantry of extra stuff, as if a crocodile preparing for hard times. Because that's how we're meant to live.

I'm not a full on Marie Kondo-er; I don't turn my T-shirts into little teepees, nor my jumpers into tiny houses. But I have become the type who donates and re-gifts stuff with wild abandon, as I know that unused, unwanted stuff carries with it the extra weight of the shoulds.

A NON-INSTAGRAM-READY HOME

'Do not spoil what you have by desiring what you have not; remember that what you now have was once among the things you only hoped for.'

Epicurus

A year ago, all I wanted in the world, *all I wanted*, was to live by the sea in my own space, so that I no longer had to be kept awake by drunken housemates clomping about at 1am inexplicably doing laundry, or crashing in at 3am like baby rhinos.

My personal favourite was the time I woke up at 4am to this sound:

Bop...bop...bop...clatter...*muffled squeak of outrage*

Bop...bop...bop...bop...clatter...*muffled exclamation of triumph*

It sounds like they're...how can they be...no, they can't be...yes, they were.

They were playing ping pong. Turns out that they owned a set that transformed the kitchen island into a table tennis match, six feet away from my sleeping head in the room above. I love a spot of table tennis, but at 4am, I wasn't feeling it.

House-sharing is stressful in that low-level, white-noise, constant-thrum kind of way. I used to exhale and do a little jig whenever I would come home to a black-windowed house, even when I was totally besotted with my housemates.

Then I got my flat and my soundtrack of seagulls screeching like wild monkeys. My forty square inches of a sea view, plus a crouching rectangle of a brown leisure centre and a muscle gym from which I'm sure I can smell the steroi...sweat. I was utterly overjoyed.

It was unfurnished, so I flipped my gaze to the next prize. All I wanted was a flat full of furniture. That was *all I wanted*. Then I would feel complete! So, I set about assembling flatpacks and sourcing vintage finds, and finally, I had an entirely furnished flat.

And then of course, I wanted to make my flat look extraordinary; like a cross between Soho House and The Frugality's Instagram feed. Never mind the fact that the houses that I long to replicate are grand dames with original stained glass, cornicing and genteel fireplaces, while my rented flat is more of an underwhelming peasant replete with peeling wallpaper, a leaking fridge and an oven that only has one setting of 'Furnace food to a crisp'.

Financially, a year ago, *all I wanted* was a little savings cushion. Then, I saved that. Then, all I wanted was a ten per cent deposit saved. Now, I have that.

So, of course, all I want is a 20 per cent deposit.

Then, I started walking down the serene wisteria-scented street I wanted to buy on. I turned my gaze to that. Now, all I want is to own a flat, on that street, with a little garden, so that I can get a cat called George (Harrison) and a cocker spaniel named Nina (Simone). That's all I want.

And once I have bought the flat, I'll no doubt start wanting to pay my mortgage off by 50.

And the cycle continues, ad infinitum. It's the property version of hedonic adaptation.

That's what we do. We shoot, we score, we bellow with triumph, then bob and weave and jump to shoot again. Indeed, psychology professor Ed Diener reported that at any one time, we tend to have six items on our wish list, and 47 per cent of us desire a bigger, better living space.

And yet, many celebrities and tycoons who could live in a cavernous mansion, deny the call of the hedonic 'more!' urge, by refusing to upsize, and stubbornly staying on their rung of the ladder. Lena Dunham lives in a modest three-bedroom house in Los Angeles, despite being worth $12 million. Zooey Deschanel could probably have bought a 12-bed while she was starring in *New Girl*, but she lived in a two-bed. Warren Buffet bought a home worth only $652,619 in today's money, which, considering he is the third richest man in the States and worth nearly $81 billion, is quite astounding.

Then, there's Tony Hsieh. The CEO of Zappos is reportedly worth a cool $840 million and yet chooses to live in a 240-square-foot trailer atop a cement car park. (Albeit a super-cool trailer park that he founded, featuring a whimsical entrance tunnel festooned with upcycled Xmas lights, a herd of llamas, plus 30 Airstreams and 'tiny houses'.)

What is *with* these extraordinarily rich folk who insist on living in ordinary houses?! I suspect because they know this: what's the point in having a house so big that you have an empty room free for a saxophone-playing Kenny G and 150 red roses to stand in it, a la Kim Kardashian's Valentine's Day gift? What's the point in having a 'present-wrapping' station the size of my kitchen, like Christina Aguilera (you can see a picture of it if you look online)? With big houses come big stress. Big cleaning. Big furnishing demands. Big amounts of family expecting to be able to come and stay for a week in your West wing.

'Dear me of a year ago...'

To counter this maximizing urge within me, I now do something on the
regular. When I find myself with a cat o' nine tails, self-flagellating for not
being further ahead, I write a letter to the me of a year ago, saying:

> Dear me of a year ago,
> In a year, you will have:
> [insert achievements, personal growth, hardscrabble knocks I have withstood]
> Isn't that incredible? Can you believe it?
> Love from future me XOXO

It reminds me how far I've come.

The letter is about remembering that once-upon-a-time, *all I wanted*, was
what I currently have. That I have made progress, even though the memory of
it has fallen out of that 'done' trapdoor in my psyche. It's worth a try, if you're
also a maximizer prone to this 'failing' feeling. The only thing you have to lose
is your own self-flagellation.

Now, I remember what I have, and how keenly I wanted it not so long
ago. But that doesn't mean I'm in starry-eyed denial. Everything in my very
ordinary rented flat needs replacing. Everything in it probably dates back to
the 1970s. Unfiltered kids walk in and exclaim 'this is so small!' while their
parents shush them.

But I don't care, because it's up on high and I can see the sorbet sunset. I can
see a flock of starlings that make their flyover on their way to murmurate on the
pier amid a blizzard of camera flashes. I love it.

One day, I will move into a place I buy, and I will remember to love
that for as long as possible too. To *not* allow my negatively biased brain, my
maximizing, my hedonic adaptation, to screw with my enjoyment of it.

And maybe I'll get myself a set that turns a kitchen island into a ping pong
table, just as a nod to where I've come from.

> 'You own twice as much rug if you're twice as *aware*
> of the rug.'
>
> Allen Ginsberg

ODES TO THE ORDINARY
An ode to local festivals

I've never been to Glastonbury. I've never even applied for a ticket.

I feel like simply saying that has set off an alarm someplace in the capital of hipsters. (I know it *was* Shoreditch. Now? No clue.) But I've never particularly wanted to go. Not badly enough to sit there click – click – clicking on a link for five hours, anyhow.

I'm a fan of a tremendously ordinary, and unbelievably cute local festival. Give me a village fete over Coachella any day.

I recently went to Swindon lit fest (affectionately known as the 'Swinge') and even though it was essentially a very 'ordinary' festival, it was my absolute favourite literature festival so far. After the chats, everyone piled back to a farmhouse B&B for sinfully creamy and cheesy food. Finished off with apple tart and a lamb attempting to eat my handbag.

The weekend previous, I had attended a very fancy, flash festival replete with celebs, designer clothes, a luxury goody bag, artisan snacks and all the trimmings.

Honestly, I enjoyed the Swinge a hundredfold more.

When I told the Swinge hosts about the theme of this book, they told me about their farmhouse 'Door Opening Ceremony' – where they cut a ribbon, prise open a door that's been shut all winter, do a conga in the wind the door lets in, play instruments and make up a poem. They also held a 'Grand Opening of the Compost Loo'. I frickin' love it.

They told me a fascinating story about a woman who wanted to go to the Amazonian rainforest to look for new species but couldn't afford it. So she grew an oasis in her tenement backyard and discovered a brand new beetle there.

Inspired by them, I am now going to treat the unrolling of very ordinary things with an extraordinary gravity of ceremony. I'm planning on buying a dishwasher, yippee, because life's too short to wash up three times a day. When it arrives, I shall wrap it in ribbon and snip it open. I'll invite some friends around for dinner on the night of its box-fresh voyage. Because...whyever not?

If a local supermarket gets an opening day, or a new line of stationery gets a launch party, why shouldn't your kids' newly decorated playroom? Buy a £1.99 lemon drizzle cake from the supermarket and have a teddy bear's picnic with tiny tea cups.

If we don't celebrate these miniscule things, they slide into insignificance, fading into the forgotten files, and within a few days, it's as if the new thing has always been there.

DEAR GENERATION RENT

Dear Generation Rent,

It's not your fault. No, really.

It's not. I know you think it is, but it's…

Not. Your. Fault.

And now I feel rather like Robin Williams' character in *Good Will Hunting.*

Renting instead of buying is now so common, that it's almost tipping over into the majority. A 2017 YouGov survey found that over four in ten 18–34-year-olds currently rent, while three in ten of 35–54-year-olds do too. Also, data shows that London now has the most expensive average rent in all of Europe. Is it any wonder big-city dwellers are struggling to squirrel away deposits?

In America, the Pew Research Center reported that 37 per cent are now renting; meteoric renting figures that haven't been witnessed since 1965. While in Australia, a recent census showed that the number of renters now equals the number who own their houses outright (rolling in at almost a third).

Sharing late into our twenties, thirties – even beyond – means we get stuck in a shared existence of psychological dishwasher-dodging warfare. Invisible tensions crisscross the air of shared houses like red lasers denoting an elaborate alarm system. Some have speculated that the low-level stress of house-sharing rushes couples into living together before they're ready (I identify, hard). In many ways, renting a space of one's own has become the new *buying* a place of one's own. There are no lasers I need to backflip to avoid in my flat, because it's just me.

The lion's share of Baby Boomers managed to get on the property ladder in their twenties simply because, back then, it was an absolute doddle to get a mortgage. Which is why they are property-rich, while Generation X-ers and Millennials are property-poor.

The chances of a 25–34-year-old on an average income owning a home has halved in the past 20 years, said 2018 research from the Institute of Fiscal Studies. In 1998, 65 per cent of that age bracket owned their own place. Now it's just 27 per cent.

But, facts such as these don't stop the Generation Rent judgers, that small but significantly annoying slice of the older generations, who spend many hours commenting on online articles, saying things like: 'We didn't have this problem back in my day! We worked hard and scrimped and saved. Must be all the vinyl and craft ale they're so fond of. Profligate!'

They have conveniently forgotten that you could often get a mortgage without a deposit 'back in their day', and that the punitive approval process of the twenty-tens didn't exist 'back in their day'. They were practically given mortgages free with their supermarket shop.

A startling 2019 report by the Financial Conduct Authority calculated the average levels of wealth for each generation, and found that in order for Millennials to catch up with Baby Boomers, they'd have to experience a 'wealth growth' of 48 per cent, year-on-year, between the ages of 20 and 36.

Which is, of course, astronomical. I don't think anyone experiences a year-on-year growth of that magnitude, unless they've been born into the silver-cradled Chanel, Walmart or Mars dynasties. 'Welcome to the world, bubba! Here, have a million dollars…'

What's more, homeowners are not necessarily happier. Some studies do bear out this societal assumption, but American research shows different. 'Contrary to popular beliefs about the "American dream"', says Professor Lyubomirsky, 'researchers have found that home owners are less happy than renters, derive more pain from ownership of their homes, and spend more time on housework and less time interacting with friends and neighbours.'

So, please accept my hug, my empathy and my solidarity Generation Rent. I am with you, I see you, and I know. Let the Gen-Rent judgers crack on with puffing out their chests. The older generations haven't a clue what it's like to get and keep a job in today's scarce, cut-throat job market, or to save the King's ransom deposits of today, so their opinion of your situation is wildly irrelevant.

The fact that it's so difficult to save a deposit now, to get a mortgage, is a direct result of the credit crunch, and nothing to do with your fondness for avo-on-toast or hot yoga. Renting deep into midlife is now supremely ordinary. Buying is becoming extraordinarily hard to do.

If you know some of the Gen-Rent judgers personally, please do toy with their predilection for side-eyeing your spending habits, and play with their tendency to disbelieve that draconian rents are to blame.

Tell them you spend £150 a week on yoga leggings or fixie bike parts, rather than save (even if this is total fiction, which it very likely is); just to watch their judgement dial swing to maximum and ding-ding-ding! To see their blood start to boil and shake.

'Hey, did I tell you that I spent £500 the other day on a tattoo on my bum? Yeah, it's so cool, I spent all of my savings on it! And I think I'm going to get a credit card to buy one of those schnoodles too (a schnauzer and poodle cross). They're only about a grand!'

Beams and bites down on some smashed avocado

Try it. It's fun!

Love,

Catherine

ORDINARY JOYS PART I

Gratitudes could alternatively be called 'ordinary joys' if the word 'gratitude' isn't flicking your switch.

From hereon in, I'm going to drop in one-pagers of 'Ordinary Joys'. With the disclaimer that they're *my* ordinary joys. You may share some with me, but oftentimes, yours will be entirely different from mine.

For instance, I love scarecrows. They make me chuckle, while other people find them creepy. My friend Kate digs it when plants climb, sneak and unfurl their way into places they're not supposed to be, as if they're trespassers reclaiming the manmade. And my cousin loses herself in the precise weighing, sifting, dusting and icing trance of baking.

I would be delighted if you could scribble down your ordinary joys in this book, as they occur to you, as they walk by you, as you feel them beside you. Because if you don't tap ordinary joys on the shoulder and say hey, they slip away into the crowd.

Books, I think, are made to be engaged with. Written in. Used. So, I invite you to please use this one by writing all over it, if that doesn't offend your book-owning sensibilities. The more defaced it is, the more honoured I will feel.

- Assembling flatpack furniture. It feels like hell in a confounding instruction manual, but once you've managed it, you feel like an actual carpenter. 'See that? I made it.' Bosh.

- Overhearing amusing, bizarre things. I recently overheard this at a luggage carousel. '[Insert budget airline] lost my suitcase, so I told them I had a WAY bigger suitcase, and now I have this humungous thing...I think I could probably sleep in it if I ever get stuck for a place to live.'

- Dusting off a forgotten retro song (Hothouse Flowers anyone?) or discovering a new one (Courteeners) that makes your heart pole-vault.

- Buying 'gifts' that you want to use yourself. (Case in point: I recently bought my niece and nephew games I loved as a kid: *Hotel*, *Buckaroo* and *Screwball Scramble*.)

- The self-satisfaction of using the last squeeze of the ketchup or shampoo and knowing you already have another one ready to roll. Adulting award: pending.

- Finally doing a non-urgent task that has been chewing at your heel for months (taking pictures to the framers, and actually hanging them).

- Babysitting for the friends with the one-year-old so that they can go to a hotel for a night. They've gotten under five hours' sleep a night for a year (true fact, the average new parents gets four hours and 44 minutes a night). They deserve it more than anyone.

- Have you ever sat and watched roofers at work? It's like a free circus act. I can barely stay upright on the pavement and yet there *they* are, balancing nimbly on a gable with a pile of tiles.

- Kitsch fish 'n' chip shop names, like 'Oh my Cod' or 'The Frying Scotsman'.

III: ORDINARY BEING

ANXIETY IS SPECTACULARLY NORMAL

Being in the thick of a panic attack and trying to behave 'normal' is like trying to act nonchalant while in the eye of a hurricane.

'No biggie.'

A small house whips past your ear

Eep.

I am a very ordinary anxious person. I'm not extraordinary. One in six of us experiences anxiety (or depression) at least once a week. So why do I feel like I'm the only one, sometimes? Because we keep our anxiety stories locked down.

- I have turned on my heel outside a supermarket, in tears, fighting an indiscernible dread building inside me.

- I have repeatedly had to tell myself that I'm not going to vomit, while a saboteur inside me yells that I'm going to vomit, while in a work meeting.

- I have sat at dinners during which my 'flight' mechanism was so activated that I actually had to hold myself on the chair, to stop my renegade body from bolting for the door.

- I have leaned against toilet walls and slowed my ragged breath to something resembling smooth, before going for a coffee with someone. How would I lift the coffee without spilling it? How would I make small talk without my voice quavering?

- A lift packed with people? I regarded those who looked bored much in the same way as I would regard an alien.

- I have stood up on hundreds of trains rather than sit opposite people, as I felt the scrutiny (read: apathy) of a stranger's gaze so keenly that it would make me hot-cheeked. My favourite train haven? Those in-between carriage pods where the rubbery floor shifts beneath your feet.

Any situation where I felt trapped, either physically or by the straitjacket of social mores, would quicken my heart into a thump (that I could have sworn was audible) and squeeze my lungs until I felt I couldn't get enough oxygen. My fingertips would tingle, my feet would become slabs of clumsy meat, my stomach would be attacked by…butterflies? Give over. More like a plague of locusts.

The secret cause of my anxiety

In an almighty plot twist, I discovered that the thing causing my anxiety was the thing I thought was curing it. Alcohol!

Alcohol, for me, was the gormless copper who features as a bit part in the detective drama. Who eventually, after a serpentine path through red herrings, 'how do they know this?' leaks and lingering glances that last a heartbeat too long, are revealed to be the secret psychopath. We thought they were helping, when they were the bad guy all along.

'Chronic stress, such as from trauma or addiction, tends to sensitize the amygdala and weaken the brain's capacity to regulate it,' says neuropsychologist Dr Hanson. The amygdala, if you recall, is the alarm system of the brain. Back when I first quit drinking, my amydala was a quivering Chihuahua who was indeed alarmed at everything.

I know alcohol was the root source of my anxiety, because with every year I put between me and my last drink (I quit in 2013) I feel calmer. And reams of studies back up my observation (one of these, carried out by UCL and Exeter University in 2018, showed that 'hangxiety' is also worse in those who are shy, like me).

But, quitting made my anxiety worse at first, particularly during social situations that involved the chest-pounding ritual of shared drinking. 'Great, is that a tray of shots dancing over towards our table?' *Grits teeth* I have literally had to cheers 'Happy Birthday!' with an empty hand as there was nothing available other than booze.

The cupcake 'cure'

Not everyone reaches for Chenin blanc or craft ale to anaesthetize anxiety, of course. For many, their reach is for food; sugar in particular.

'Unfortunately your brain doesn't come with a user manual,' says Dr Korb. 'We don't have a car dashboard with warning lights to show us what's going on.

So we often mistake anxiety for hunger, given hunger often prompts distress (hence "hangry").' You learn that eating a cupcake helps you feel less stressed. 'It changes your physiology and pushes you towards more parasympathetic activity, which is when our brain and body relaxes.'

Cue: the subsequent eating of more cupcakes.

And it's no flamin' wonder we're sugar fiends, given that historically it has been such a fast-lane to energy and fat, which was something our ancestors lacked. Sugar was rare, unless they were rich as royalty. Regrettably, our slowcoach brains have still not caught up with the fact that sugar is now exceedingly common, in the shape of sugar cereal, sugar juices, sugar bars, sugar smoothies...sugar rushes are now ordinary, but our brains still ring-a-ding-ding for them like they're *extra*ordinary. 'Gimme!' they holler.

I may as well worry about rhinos

I now have many, many go-to anxiety cures. On Big Days, I halve my caffeine intake. I use calming essential oil roll-ons, sniffing lavender like my life depends on it. I give myself double the amount of time to get ready. And much more besides...

1. **I bring my rational brain online**
   In order to highlight the fact that it's my irrational amygdala telling myself I am about to forget how to say words when I step foot on the stage, I bring my prefrontal cortex into the room, by telling my amygdala this:

   'Given I have never, ever forgotten how to say words, or upturned a meeting table, vomited randomly, or collapsed, or whatever else poppycock you are saying, I am now going to worry about something else that has also never happened. That a herd of rhinos will burst through the wall.'

   I then amuse myself by thinking about other catastrophic scenarios that have *also never happened*, say that the person I'm having a meeting with will turn into a vampire, or that the bus will start to fly. It works, for me.

2. **I box breathe**
   In for four, hold for four, out for four, hold for four. Because when I'm spinning out, I'm invariably holding my breath, like that will help matters. This activates your parasympathetic nervous system, the opposite of 'fight or flight', or in other words, it calms you the frig down. Where the body goes, the brain will start to follow.

It's like three-time Olympic gold medallist Kristin Armstrong says, 'When everything is moving and shifting, the only way to counteract chaos is stillness. When things feel extraordinary, strive for ordinary. When the surface is wavy, dive deeper for quieter waters'.

3. I exercise five times a week

When I don't, my system gets clogged with adrenaline and cortisol; sweating on a seafront run, sun salutations on the mat or a fierce front crawl literally flush these stressors from my system.

4. I use the big picture hack

Neuroscientist Dr Korb says it's really useful to ask yourself to remember the big picture. 'There's this great study where they took participants and told them "you have five minutes to come up with a presentation"', says the author of *The Upward Spiral*. 'Which obviously provoked stress.'

'But they discovered that if they then asked the participants to think about what's important in their life and why, just before they went on stage, it reduced their cortisol and thus the intensity of their stress.' Presumably, it reminded them that the next five minutes, and what the researchers think of their hotchpotch presentation, is miniscule in the grand scheme of things.

5. ASMR

I once caught a dear friend watching ASMR videos in my bedroom and was convinced, given the way she'd just snapped her laptop shut in fright, that she'd been watching porn.

'I didn't want you to think I'm weird,' she tentatively said, shrinking with shame as she opened her screen to reveal a video of a twentysomething whispering about working in a coffee shop, stroking velvet scrunchies, tapping her nails against things and unpeeling stickers. We both sat there for five minutes, inexplicably hypnotized. 'I get it,' I said, practically drooling by the end. I've been hooked ever since.

ASMR stands for Autonomous Sensory Meridian Response. It's like feelgood fireflies dancing in the centre of your brain. It's utterly delicious. Don't knock it until you've tried it.

Having arguments in my head

I know when I need to up my anti-anxiety defences with some nourishing self-parenting when one particular thing happens. I start having arguments in my head with people. Constantly imagining ways people could have a pop at me, reasons they may be annoyed with me, and constructing sentences with which to defend myself, or coax them into liking me once more.

I imagine the thwack, thwack, thwack back-and-forth of arguments that haven't happened yet, and are highly unlikely to ever happen in my lifetime. She'll say, then I'll say, then she'll say…I really have to catch myself and pull myself out of the pre-emptive strike scriptwriting.

'It's your brain's negative bias acting up,' explains Dr Rick Hanson, author of *Hardwiring Happiness*. 'Re-playing a run-in with your neighbours, and almost building a case against them like a lawyer.'

Perhaps this is the fall-out of a combative home life when I was a teen, or a critical father, or my drinking causing more skirmishes than was normal way-back-when. But actually, I think it's just a common precursor to anxiety. Your brain starts building a bunker and assembling tinned food, in order to prepare for the zombie apocalypse. An apocalypse that will never happen.

The irony is, as soon as acute anxiety goes away, we tend to drop the things that made it go away in the first place. Author Michael Foley wrote about how he recovered from panic attacks in his book *Embracing the Ordinary: lessons from the champions of everyday life*.

'I did a meditation exercise every day. The stress symptoms began to ease and there was an unexpected side-effect – the view that I was looking out upon, the noisy, littered railway line behind my home, an estate agent's nightmare, gradually became a place of wonder. The honking of passing trains was as lyrical as the cries of wild geese flying overhead. The rampant Japanese knotweed that had colonized the embankments was a manifestation of the glory and resourcefulness of nature.'

Remarkable. And yet, he stopped. 'So I have been a committed meditator ever since? Of course not. As soon as the stress symptoms went away I gave up the meditating.'

I have to remember *not to stop*.

Even now, I always feel slightly on edge and like I'm about to get into trouble. I rush my use of public bathrooms for fear I will open the door and find someone standing there, tutting that I dared to wash and thoroughly dry my hands.

Anxiety is why I have to go to the loo three times before bed. It's why I feel stricken if I can't book an aisle seat at the cinema or theatre. It's why splitting a bill, which doesn't seem to faze other people, makes me want to hide under the table.

Anxiety still lives within me, and likely always will do, like a tiny silver sphere sitting within an arcade machine awaiting its pinball release, but I know what to do now when it goes pow! When it cannonballs up to my brain, shoots to the ends of my fingers, and speeds to my organs, my heart, my lungs, my stomach, my feet. Something I didn't know for the longest time.

What works for you will be as unique as your thumb print. Investigate. Try everything. Knowledge is power. And remember, it's utterly, fantastically commonplace for your brain to be like a quivering Chihuahua. Remember the survival of the most negative? It's just your brain trying to save your skin. It's up to us to reassure our brains that death is not upon us. To tell it that everything is A-OK.

ODES TO THE ORDINARY

An ode to where the wild things are

We underestimate the therapeutic power of the countryside. Even an ordinary woodland walk (which featured no hot tubs, waterfalls or silky-sand beaches) has the power to improve our mood by 88 per cent, one study by mental health charity, Mind, found*

There's a reason why nature programmes have seen such an upsurge in popularity recently (take the galactic success of *Planet Earth II*) and that's because, in diabolical times such as right *now*, people find comfort where the wild things are.

We long to be outside and barefoot, particularly in tempestuous times. Professor Cregan-Reid brings up 'biophilia'; a theory coined by biologist and naturalist Edward O Wilson, to describe human gravitation and attraction to other living organisms. 'Our bodies crave to be outdoors doing things they recognize as simulations of hunting and gathering,' says Cregan-Reid.

He goes on to to point out studies which show that people recuperate more quickly after operations when they can see green space. 'The human eye is adapted to see more shades of green than any other colour,' he adds. 'Green is like the room temperature of our visual spectrum, since it's right in the middle, and is the colour our brain has to do the least processing to see.'

Even when we *think* we love being in cities, given it's exciting and fun, it's like a five-year-old who believes they prefer cordial to water, says Cregan-Reid. 'They're just hooked on the sugar buzz. It doesn't mean it's good for them. It's in our DNA to want – to expect – natural environments.'

Ordinary, for us, is the countryside. Cities are bamboozling to our bodies, while the rural is soothing. Only giving our bodies The City is like giving a child a giant, airport-sized candy bar and allowing them to eat it unmonitored. Remember the point about cities having sprung up at 4.59pm, if the existence of our species were 9 to 5? That.

So, it's really important to allow our minds, bodies, and bare feet to feel even the unexceptional grass/ sand/ soil of our local forest, park, or beach. It may not be a photo opportunity, the water may be freezing rather than swimmable, and it may tip it down, but your mind and body will still thank you for it. They don't care how 'extra' it is – they just want to be there.

---

* Interestingly, the study also found that a stroll in a shopping centre only saw a 45 per cent hike in mood. This could be why 'forest bathing' is more popular than 'chain store strip-light bathing'.

MID-RANGE SELF-ESTEEM

There's a modern idea that floor-to-ceiling, extraordinary self-esteem is desirable. Hmmm. Actually, research shows that those who rate themselves the most highly (generally narcissists) are unlikeable, risky, even dangerous individuals.

Nicholas Emler, a professor of social psychology, has long sought to puncture this idea that we should all want to be puffed-up.

He says that high self-esteem is, 'very unlikely to be the all-purpose social vaccine that some have supposed it to be. Indeed, it seems to have some disadvantages.' Those with bulletproof self-esteem tend to be prejudiced against ethnic minorities, reject social influence and engage in risky pursuits.

Professor Emler thinks that the common usage of put-downs such as 'big-headed', 'smug' and 'boastful' serves a purpose. 'These reflect the wisdom of culturally accumulated experience,' is his slam-dunk parting shot.

This is comforting, because self-doubt is like my spine. It is an unavoidable part of my anatomy. I have spent years thinking this is a bad thing, and trying to remove my spine, but I have now realized it is simply a part of me, and so I need to work with it.

'What do you like about me?' was a question I frequently asked in my twenties, which seemed cocksure and narcissistic at the time, but was because my self-esteem was a malnourished kitten which needed hand-feeding by others. I found it inconceivable that people liked me and was genuinely curious as to why they did. Just as I was genuinely curious as to why on earth people would like ice-water baths, or insects as a delicacy.

So, it's comforting to know that armoured-tank self-esteem is actually not something we should long for. My ordinary, average self-esteem will do just fine, as will yours.

ODES TO THE ORDINARY
An ode to lie-ins

I have a morbid fascination for those 'day in the life of' articles in magazines, that show perfectly blow-dried people perched on the edges of geometrically laid-out desks. Have you noticed they always, always get up before 7am? Usually to meditate and drink hot, lemony water.

I've never read about one who rolls out of bed between 8am and 9am, like me, and snuffles around for the strongest coffee they can find, like a pig hunting truffles. I think if a 'day in the life of' person admitted to getting up at 8.30am, the page their diary is published upon would spontaneously burst into indignant flames.

We're constantly being told that less sleep equals more success. There's Marissa Mayer, Yahoo's CEO, who allegedly gets four hours a night, or Richard Branson who reportedly gets five. But this largely appears to be based on hearsay. Who knows whether it's actually true, or whether it's something manufactured by the sleep propaganda machine.

Insert business titan and machine spits out low number of hours slept per night

The invisible ink narrative says that ordinary commoners need sleep (scorn level of tone: maximum) because they're pussies, whereas entrepreneurial comets even *sleep* more efficiently, because if you're not up by sunrise, then what the Dickens are you doing with your life?!

Yet, there's a behemoth of a whistleblower calling time on this sleep-starving myth. In a now-infamous wake-up call, Arianna Huffington, founder of *The Huffington Post*, collapsed from sleep deprivation, smacked her head on the corner of her desk, and woke up in a pool of blood, having broken her cheekbone and sliced her eyelid open.

Arianna then went onto write *Thrive*, about how she has gone from battling through on three to four hours sleep, to giving a TED talk on *How to succeed? Get more sleep*. She even ran a competition for a winner to spend a night in her bedroom; her 'sleep sanctuary' in which the rules are that devices and pets are replaced by candles and books of poetry.

'The need for eight hours' sleep is evolutionary,' she told the *Guardian*. 'It's not negotiable. If we ignore that need, we pay a huge price in every aspect of our health and cognitive performance.' She adds, 'When I'm sleep deprived, I tend to focus on what is not working rather than what is working.' Every logical person identifies with this. Our fears become bigger, our problems insurmountable, our dreads blacker somehow, on a bad night's sleep.

As a result of all the 'sleep less, do more!' propaganda, I've tried valiantly to be an early riser. I've sometimes done it, by accident, by way of too-thin curtains, or jet lag. And felt very smug about it. But no matter what I do, I gradually zzz back into my 8am-ish rising time.

If you're the same, listen up. It's just science. It's your DNA, rather than a sign you will never rule the world. Whether you are an owl like me, or an extreme lark like all of the 'day in the life of' ~~fibbers~~ people, is determined by our DNA, said a genetic study of nearly 90K people.

Only having six hours sleep a night, voluntarily, is not a sign that you are tipped for supreme greatness, it's not an *extraordinary* feat ... it's an omen of an oncoming nervous breakdown.

Sleep. We need it. Let's not sleep-shame each other. And, remember this. Donald Trump only sleeps between 1am and 5am, he claims, in *Trump: think like a billionaire*.

Schools of thought posit that maybe *that's* why he's apparently so hellbent on global decimation. (Personally, I think he's been sent from an alien race that wants to ensure our ultimate destruction.)

ANGER DOES NOT MAKE YOU A 'BAD' PERSON

If you move in yogic, or hippy, or similar circles, there tends to be a lot of chat of shuffling off the mortal coil of anger: 'I have moved beyond anger and detached from my ego,' is something I've heard. While someone self-satisfied once preached to me, 'Anger is a luxury I can no longer afford, so I just don't go there, you shouldn't either'.

Oh deep irony, that it made me want to flick her on the forehead. It just feels so disingenuous, when people claim to have transcended even the smallest pulse of irritation.

The 'enlightened' make extraordinary claims of living an anger-free existence, while the ordinary among us, those peasants whose minds have not clambered to a higher plane of serenity, experience the throttle of anger on average four times a day, says anger expert Michael Fisher.

Anger is not a naughty emotion to be erased, or the preserve of the dumbass dharma-less. It is spectacularly normal. And anybody who claims not to feel it, is either a liar, in denial, or perhaps even a psychopath. Experiencing anger is not bad in and of itself; it's the volcanic eruption of it that can be.

Healthily venting anger by punching a pillow, or running hard, or inserting pins into an app voodoo doll, is not necessarily bad if it stops you from being a knob in real life. Whereas those who deny anger's existence, or stuff it down can often find that it leaks out, in passive-aggressive pops. Or it turns inwards.

Anger can be repurposed into comedic gold, providing the pricelessly acerbic rants of Billy Connolly, George Carlin, or Ali Wong (angry female comedians are generally conspicuous by their absence, because men are allowed to be angry, while women are not).

In its worthiest form, anger serves an important social purpose, in rising up against injustice. Imagine if Rosa Parks had rolled over and given up her seat on that fateful day in 1955. Or if Stormé DeLarverie had not pushed back against police and sparked the Stonewall Riots, regarded as the catalyst of the gay rights movement in the late sixties. Or if Jan Rose Kasmir, she of the iconic 'The Flower and the Bayonet' picture, had not had the guts to go and face down the barrel of a gun to place a chrysanthemum stem inside it.

Or if Russell Crowe *Gladiator* had not...hold up, that last one's not real.

Anger can often serve as a unignorable clue that you are doing something, or spending time with someone, or working someplace, that you should leave behind. It can battery-pack you away from bad relationships or situations, into safety. Being consistently angry is your nervous system saying: my boundaries are being crossed, I'm unhappy, and sod this for a game of soldiers.

When anger malfunctions

But personally, my history of anger was nowhere near as just or reliable an alarm system. It was an offshoot of self-loathing. And it was because I was so freakin' tired – and hungover – all of the time.

My system malfunctioned and my drinking created an anger within me that was akin to a wasp nest. Every morning I would wake up feeling rancid and the internal nest would start to thrum. A wasp would sting someone if they accidentally bumped me on the tube. Another would chase after a colleague if they forgot me on the tea run. Another wasp would terrorize a friend if they wouldn't lend me money, because I felt entitled to be bailed out (having spent all of my disposable income in a sticky-carpeted nightclub).

It was exhausting. And obviously, entirely pointless, rather than a righteous thrust against injustice.

When I sobered up, I learned that anger can often just be a Halloween mask. Once you remove the scary facade, what sits beneath it is often sadness, fear, grief; something much less shouty. I discovered that the best way to avoid drinking 'at' whatever person scared or saddened me, was to really allow myself to explore and feel whatever the mask was disguising.

Once you learn to retract the defensive spikes, remove the mask and allow yourself to be emotionally vulnerable, the real emotion reveals itself.

A wise friend of mine recently said her therapist told her, 'People who are shouting generally really want to cry'. A scarlet-faced road rage rant is often because whatever happened scared the bejesus out of you.

I love what Jonah Hill said when a troll called him a 'fat nerd' on Instagram. 'Anger is just sadness held in too long. I'm here for you dude.'

Little boys in particular are often encouraged to have the emotional intelligence of rocks. They're taught that anger is their only acceptable negative emotion.

Don't believe me? Put a boy in a playground and ask him to start sobbing or talking about his feelings. The result would be the bullied, teased kid from the start of *About a Boy* (who later transforms into a snarky kid with expensive trainers, which is the socially accepted version of a boy). It's a travesty.

Psychologist Michael Addis put it beautifully in his book *Invisible Men*. 'A man's masculinity is measured in large part by his ability to make his public accomplishments widely seen and heard, while keeping his inner life silent and invisible.' Which he says leads, among other things, to higher levels of drug and alcohol use in men.

When I do let anger poison-dart my tongue, when my conscience is chewing me out for an outburst, it's simple; I just apologize. I've apologized to two people in the past 24 hours; my brother and a call-centre worker. For being an accidental twat.

Admission of wrong-doing does not make you a bad person. On the contrary, it makes you a good one. And anger is essentially ordinary. Those who claim never to feel it? Are kidding themselves.

ODES TO THE ORDINARY
An ode to yoga

People who *don't* do yoga think yoga is relaxing – because it's relaxing. Baha!

Unless you're in a sleepy Hatha class, most yoga is fearsomely difficult. Yoga actually relaxes you because it's *not relaxing*.

'As a neuroscientist,' says Dr Korb, 'despite my initial incredulity, I came to realize that yoga works not because the poses are relaxing, but because they are stressful. It is your attempts to remain calm during this stress that creates yoga's greatest neurobiological benefit.'

Breathing through discomfort is a yogic superpower. Learning to smoothe your breath from rasping to rolling in a savage lizard pose, even though your hip is screaming. Stilling your mind in a wobbly dancer's pose, despite feeling like you're about to tumble down in a tangle of limbs.

I recently went to a hygienist for an intensive teeth-cleaning session. 'Hold up your hand if it becomes too much,' she said, at the beginning. I didn't hold up my hand. At the end she said, incredulous, 'I've gotta ask, do you use some de-sensitizing toothpaste or something, because there were some moments there that must have been really uncomfortable, yet you didn't ask me to stop.'

There was no special toothpaste. Only my extensive experience of two things; getting sober and practising yoga. I have now learned to stay still through discomfort and trust that *I will not die.*

Dr Korb is also a big fan of the classes that incorporate the 'clench and then de-clench' tactic just before Savasana (otherwise known as 'corpse'; the final pose). 'We don't necessarily know that our fingers are tight or our jaw is tense until we tense them and then un-tense them,' he says.

Give it a whirl and see how good it feels. Clench – de-clench – aaaah.

NOBODY GETS 100 PER CENT GOOD REVIEWS

Not every friend, date, work contact or family member will want you, no matter how freaking fabulous you are. But rejection is just a re-direction. It's like a satnav that takes you around a snarl of a traffic jam, or a closed road, or a wrong turn. So, even though your journey time gets longer and you whack the steering wheel, and it smarts and you swear a little, you will end up finding the things meant for you instead.

Rejection is often very little to do with you. 'People are in stories you have no idea about,' someone wise once told me. Yet, when we're rejected, our self-loathing and narcissism dovetail until we make it intensely personal. 'I'm the piece of shit at the centre of the universe' as the recovery saying goes. Everything is about me, but also: everyone hates me. The moon orbits me, but it can't bear to look at my face. I'm hated, but discussed by all.

It's that feeling when you walk into a room and two people stop talking, and you assume that they *must have been* talking about how abominable you are. Because what else could it be? (Many, many things.)

Up until the past few years, when people ended a relationship with me, I would stalk them for 'closure', as I liked to call it. I would want to know why. What I had done; what I hadn't done. But now I see that their reasons are none of my business. I don't need to know them.

I no longer hound people for closure, but I do make sure I spend some time with a dog after any kind of rejection, since it's proven (in a 2012 study entitled 'Man's best friend') that a dog can inoculate against the fall-out of social exclusion.

When you think back to rejections from yonks back, don't they nearly always lead to something better? Well then. Rejection tends to be the universe's protection.

Coping with bad reviews

One way that the writer Matt Haig deals with the inevitable bad reviews, is to look at William Shakespeare's rating on GoodReads, which at the time of going to press, was an underwhelming 3.87. Yup, less than four stars out of five for the most celebrated writer of all time. Insert 'wah-wah-wahhhh' sound effect. Inspired by this, I started doing the same thing.

Whenever I got pelted by fruit, I would take comfort in looking up writers whose words I luxuriate in (David Mitchell, Chimamanda Ngozi Adichie, Celeste Ng) and checking out their bad reviews. I felt a swell of relief that they too had been chewed and spat out by critics.

It sounds like I'm slowing down next to a car crash, but I wasn't rolling my window down in schadenfreude, gleefully pointing at the slurs in one-star Amazon reviews. What I was actually doing, was reading those damning reviews and thinking 'how very dare they trash Celeste Ng's crackling, perfect prose.'

I was reminding myself that all writers, all *people*, no matter who they are, and what they write or do, have to put up with the odd wazzock toilet-papering their house, or doing a shouty 'mediocre!' drive-by.

And that applies to everyone, whether your trade is making soy lattes, delivering presentations on climate change, or sewing skirts. Ain't everyone gonna like what you do. It's just life. An inevitable side effect. Nobody gets 100 per cent, or a perfect five stars, once you usher your work into the public realm (unless it's your family doing the reviewing).

So, you're in an arena...

I recently experienced a battering of 'You suck' on a comments section. (If you parrot 'don't read the comments' at me, I will point out that everyone reads the comments.) It wounded me, deeply.

For comfort, a reader directed me to Brené Brown's 'Why your critics aren't the ones who count' speech. Brené talks about those who share their work in public, or at all, with anybody, as being in 'an arena'. She talks about how the vast majority of the arena are cheerleaders, but we choose to zero in on, and stare at, and attempt to win over our fiercest critics. And by doing so, we're doing a disservice to our cheerleaders. I was failing to appreciate my supporters.

As are you, whenever you choose to recall all the times that people have said bad things to you, rather than putting the good things up in lights. It's entirely natural to do this, given we now know that the negative tattoos itself on our brain, but you can turn even the dodgiest 'Mum' scroll tattoo into a work of art, if you overlay it with some badass ink.

By not honouring the people standing up, and instead staring at the trolls sitting down and tapping heckles into their phones (rather than saying it to my face, never to my face), I was committing a crime. It was the equivalent of saying 'oh, this old thing, it's a bag o' shite' when somebody says 'nice outfit' to us, which is the equivalent of knocking a gift cupcake out of somebody's hand and smushing it on the floor beneath our heel.

By homing in on our critics, rather than giving the full beam to our cheerleaders, we are doing that too. Nobody gets a universal thumbs-up, with the possible exceptions of Michelle Obama or Gandhi, and even they get their fair share of stick. To wit, here are some real reviews from the interweb...

Enter Graham on Michelle Obama: *'This wo-man is not inspirational... Since she got pally with James Corden, and his ilk of supposed comedians... Millennial loving, all-caring superficiality and stinking rich talentless wife of a President. A self promotional celebrity bargain bin book for those who love the Kardashians and that self-absorbed sort of nobodys'* (one star).

And Paviter on Gandhi: *'Dreadful book! I got this book a while ago. Ungripping, uninspriringly written. About a pathetic little mans peaceful protests!!! Awful English, extremely inconcise. What an unispirational, weak, annoying excuse of a man'* (one star).

(Apologies for the spelling and grammar; reviews have been printed as they appeared online ;-)

Try looking up the people you admire the most and finding their critics, whether it's a basketball player, a biologist or a fashion designer. This will show you exactly what I mean. Everyone has their section of haters. It's crazy ordinary to have them.

What your rejectionists are really saying

Nonetheless, I don't think it's the answer to totally ignore criticism.

My bad reviews tend to have common themes. That I'm middle-class (guilty as charged), that I'm self-absorbed (guilty as charged), that I'm writing from a female perspective (this is unavoidably true given my genitals and cis alignment), that I'm rich (which my friends think is hilarious), or that my research/stats are dubious (when I list the sources faithfully and painstakingly in the back of every book).

One reviewer said my book was all 'Jamaica inn and Mr Big and skiing trips'. She's clearly confused me with Carrie Bradshaw given I have literally never experienced, let alone written about, these things.

When I break it down, what are they really saying? That I need to somehow migrate classes, or change my gender, or that they bought a memoir thinking there would be no personal stories, or that they don't like my stats/ studies given it contradicts something they believe, and thus have chosen to completely ignore the hefty Sources section? Or that they think I'm Carrie Bradshaw.

Dig beneath the bad review and source what they're really saying, and whether it's something you want to change. Maybe your parent calls you selfish for growing healthy boundaries, saying no and no longer bending over backwards. (It's a generational divide, those born from the sixties onwards usually get boundaries and embrace them, while those born before mostly don't. Boundaries are the emotional equivalent of quinoa.) Do you really want to change the thing they're asking you to change? Or is 'the thing' otherwise known as – growth?

Having said that, there are also constructive bad reviews, and I am well up for those. In fact, I once changed the actual text in a book (for reprints) thanks to an intelligent and quite right reviewer. Sometimes, when you sift out the grit, there's a golden nugget or three that is worth keeping; that could make you a better person.

Not everyone is going to like you. And if they do, it's likely you're contorting yourself into all sorts of people-pleasing shapes in order to be liked. And when you are constantly saying yes to everyone else, or yes to drinks you don't want, or yes to people trying to matchmake you when you're perfectly content single, or yes to nights out you don't wanna go on, or yes to favours you don't have time to do, you are saying no to yourself.

Nobody gets an all-auditorium standing ovation. No-bod-y. There's always a few scowling at the back. Let them. They're in everyone's auditorium. Even Gandhi's.

'If everyone likes you, you're not doing it right.'

Bette Davis

ODES TO THE ORDINARY

An ode to homegrown mini-breaks

I recently went for a three-night mini-break in exotic Kent. I came back just as rested and just as holidayed – scratch that, *more so* – than I would have done had I flown to the South of France.

Why? It cost about half the price. It took me two hours – total – to get there. I didn't have to fiddle around downloading apps to check in online, or print a boarding pass, when nobody has a printer anymore.

I didn't have to get injections, or get to the train station two hours before, or deal with budget airline delays, or get a wallopingly expensive taxi the other side. On my return, I had no sunburn to treat, or insect bites to try not to itch, or jet lag to recover from, or stowaway sand that scatters and hides.

The joy of a mini-break is all about being released from the daily toil of the laundry, the food buying, the dishwasher – the 32 things bleeping around your immediate vicinity that need doing at some point, like tiny red attackers in a Nintendo game.

And we don't need to fly anyplace to experience that release.

ODES TO THE ORDINARY
An ode to cleaning

There's a reason why Martha Stewart goes viral cleaning ovens. It's why Mrs Hinch has become a British sensation, she of two million Instagram followers, who apparently doesn't do much more than post pictures of her gleaming windows and a toilet bowl you could eat your lunch off.

It's not about the cleaning itself; it's about the decompression the cleaning/de-cluttering has on your mental health. The natural high you get from having pride in and ordering your immediate environment. As the adage goes, if you want an insight into someone's inner life, look at two things: their home and phone.

I experienced an emotional shock recently. After a long hard bawl and about four hours on the phone, I spent most of the next day spring cleaning my flat. I didn't plan it. It just happened. I started cleaning and de-cluttering and couldn't stop. My mind told me what to do. It told me I needed it. Five hours later I had a sparkling flat and a much happier mind.*

Cleaning is an act of self-respect. I do it because I love living someplace fragrant that doesn't have a bin that could be used as a biological weapon, or bits on the lino that stick to bare feet. I do it because I deserve to slip into clean sheets once a week, and so do you. I do it now, even if nobody is coming over, because I do it for myself.

I used to think my cleaning was procrastination but it's actually that your environment is an extension of your brain, and if your surroundings feel messy, your brain does too. A disordered environment is more likely to lead to dysfunctional choices.

A fascinating 2007 Harvard study found that how you perceive the cleaning has a dramatic effect. The study took 84 hotel maids and told half of them in great detail about how the act of cleaning rooms was 'good

---

* I left the oven though. I'm not a masochist.

exercise' that could improve their fitness. The other half weren't told this. Within a month, the half who now believed cleaning was great for their physical health showed reductions in blood pressure, body fat and waist-to-hip ratio. The remaining half saw no change in their body.

It's when cleaning mounts up that it begins to cause distress, I find. Now, I do something very simple. If I see something gross, like a dusty plug socket, a manky mirror or a vegetable drawer growing a new species, I just blast it – then and there. Micro-cleaning, like the gratitudes, is the way forward. Fifteen minutes a day. I know people who do it while the adverts are on.

Living underneath your sink, there is a very ordinary and insanely effective mental health overhaul sitting waiting for you. You'll find it within a tangerine-bright spray bottle.

WE ARE NOT UNFLAPPABLE
ANDROIDS

We have a national aversion to vulnerability, much like queue-jumpers. I wonder if one day it will be possible to encase ourselves in a second skin that looks just like us, but shrouds sadness or pain. We'll press a button and voom, we'll drop into an escape-hatch and allow our alt-self to handle the predicament; while we do our socially awkward emoting in a virtual reality tunnel away from prying eyes.

Indeed, this sounds like utter fantasy, but it's not as outrageous as you may think. 'We live in a world in which genetic code may soon be as editable as HTML,' says Professor Cregan-Reid. 'Therefore it might be tempting for science to muck about with our emotions, removing undesirable ones. But without unpleasant physical and emotional states, empathy, curiosity and fascination are lost.' We need the wobbles, in order to retain our humanity, essentially.

I've needed to learn how to be vulnerable in public now that I don't drink. Because drinking is actually very similar to the Spock-like alt-self. It drops a veil, it turns the volume down, and even though it may feel as if it throws your shutters open and allows people in, it actually increases the distance between you. It's a lot like how you feel like you love everyone while on MDMA, or that you're King o' the World on cocaine. You can tell that drunk vulnerability is faux because when the drug wears off, so does your newfound bond with whoever.

Crying in front of someone when you're sober is a lot, lot harder than crying when you're smashed. I've wept to the guy at Chicken Cottage before (they were out of fried chicken). Crying sober feels much more intimate and ultimately exposing, much like sober sex.

MY VULNERABILITY IN OCTOBER 2013

I am a little over a month sober and going for my first sober pub lunch with my best friend Sam, my boyfriend and her family. I have known Sam since I was 11 and she probably knows me better than any other friend.

I feel alarmed about the meal, but don't tell anyone. Must hide vulnerability and pretend you're OK, right? As soon as we sit down, with the bar in eyeline, the concoction of the smell, sight and prospect of booze triggers a piston-pounding-heart, breath-holding panic attack. I feel like I'm going to be sick.

I get up and leave in tears. Sam dashes after me and asks if I'm OK. I'm mortified. 'I have the beginning of a migraine,' I tell her. It's the ailment closest to how I actually feel, which is like I can't walk, eat, see; basically be anywhere but lying down in a dark room.

My ability to be vulnerable, even with Sam who has known me for 22 years, is zero.

MY VULNERABILITY IN JUNE 2019
During today's run, I tripped (over thin air, klutz 'til I die) and hand/knee-planted in front of a gaggle of builders.

2013-me would have sprung up, 'I'm OK honest!' and sprinted away, furious at myself for exhibiting imperfection.

But 2019-me laughs, sobs and sits on the floor for five minutes collecting myself, inspecting my grazed hands and knees, before limping off.

Somewhere along the way, the kid in us that howls hard when we fall, is taught to bounce up and pretend to be OK. We need to un-learn that and say 'Hey, I'm not OK.' Because being not OK is indeed – OK.

Had I done two things in October 2013, I probably wouldn't have had to leave the gastropub in tears. a) given myself permission to leave at any point. It was the 'I must not leave!' pressure that ultimately caused the claustrophobic spin-out b) told Sam how I was feeling about my first sober pub meal and asked for support.

By allowing myself to feel how I was feeling, by not 'NONONO' pushing away that feeling, I would have felt it less acutely. The feeling likely would have passed through me like a movie ghost – in, shudder, out, gone – rather than bearing down on me like a monster that I felt I had to flee from. I now know this. I didn't then.

Emotions are not Bloody Mary

I was recently stood beside a stage at an event, waiting to go up in front of an audience with a panel of four other people. Three of the four were clearly nervous.

But when I said, 'I'm nervous, how's about you guys?' they maintained they were fine. It was only afterward that they admitted they too had been nervous. It's as if we think naming an emotion can unleash something terrible, just as chanting 'Bloody Mary' in a mirror makes her spectre appear.

The reality is that naming an emotion is more of a protective spell, an exorcism, than a Satanic summoning. A willingness to be vulnerable, to drop the android 'computer says no emote' pretence, loosens the grip whatever-negative-emotion has on you.

If you imagine yourself enclosed in a fist, simply saying 'I'm nervous,' or 'I'm scared' or 'I'm sad' means the fist unfurls a little. You're still being held by the emotion, but you're sitting on its palm, rather than crunched in between its fingers, fighting to breathe. The emancipation of such 'naming' techniques is well documented by dozens of psychological studies.

'Simply naming an emotion is powerful,' confirms neuroscientist Dr Korb, 'because the mere act of naming uses language, which brings the prefrontal cortex (PFC) online. The PFC can then reduce the intensity of the emotion.'

It's why one of the first rules of hostage negotiation school is to ask the hostage-taker to name how they feel. Simply using an adjective to pin the emotion down, means they are less possessed by its sway.

We assume people will like us less, if we reveal our vulnerabilities, but the irony is, it only makes them like us more. Vulnerability is immensely likeable.

I gravitate MORE towards the anxious, bumbling and tongue-tied at any party, rather than the ones swaggering, braying and holding court.

In fact, Dr Korb thinks that vulnerability and gratitude are two sides of the same coin. 'In order to identify what we're really grateful for, we have to accept our vulnerability,' he says. 'To acknowledge that things could have – still might – go a different way.' Which can be unsettling.

We think vulnerability is weakness, without realizing that the chinks in our armour, the cracks, are where, to paraphrase Leonard Cohen, the light gets in.

ODES TO THE ORDINARY

An ode to stressful times that become good stories

Whenever you're next inside the eye of a stressful storm, repeat after me: 'One day this will be a story I tell people.'

A few years back, I was travelling alone from Mexico to Florida. As I stood in the line for customs, it occurred to me that I had seen many films in which lone women had acted as drug mules. I tried to make myself look as innocent as possible, which always has the opposite effect on my errant face.

Then, they started showing a video of a dog finding a carrot in a bag, and the carrot-bearer getting into trouble for bringing farm produce across the border. Meep. I had a rogue apple jostling around in my bag.

I started to sweat profusely. So of course, by the time I reached the customs official, they took one look at me and marched me to the back office where I was questioned as to why I was in Mexico, who I was bridesmaid for, how long had I known her, could I show them pictures?

After this rapid-fire round of questions, which were supremely simple, and yet hard to answer given they were being barked at me by an emotionless Robocop (who I felt sure they simply plugged in and charged like an electric car overnight), they finally let me go.

But no, I still had one more stage to go. As I exited the interview room section, I was faced with another customs official with an x-ray machine.

'Is there anything in your bag that can hurt me Miss?' he asked me.

No, I assured him.

'What about any drugs?'

Definitely not, I stuttered.

'So what *is* in your bag? What will I find if I open it up?' he asked.

My mind went totally blank.

What was in my bag?

Must give a specific answer, due to journalistic training.

'Er...um...shampoo! And...dresses!' I replied. And then I told him about the stowaway apple. He laughed and binned it.

What was a bum-clenchingly stressful moment, has become my 'shampoo and dresses' story. Things that are not necessarily fun in the moment, later turn into precious anecdotes.

WHEN SUNNY-SIDE-UP PSYCHOLOGY GOES TOO FAR

There's an amazing YouTube video of a bear and a goat, called 'Brené Brown on Empathy'. If you can, go and watch it now. I'll wait here.

For those who can't watch it, here's an ever-so-brief description. Brené Brown is outlining the difference between empathy and sympathy using the animals. Empathy fuels connection, while sympathy drives disconnection, she says. 'Empathy is feeling with people,' explains research professor Brown.

The goat represents sympathy, while the bear is a boss at empathy.

'Rarely, if ever, does an empathic response begin with "At least"', says Brown. 'At least' is the preserve of the sympathetic, which seems good, but it's undermining the difficult emotion a person is sharing with you.

'At least you *have* a marriage,' says the goat, having been told a marriage is failing.

'At least you know you can get pregnant,' says the goat, after news of a miscarriage.

A friend recently confided in me that she felt blue about her 'career going sideways'. In response, I gave her an 'At least!' laundry list of infuriatingly upbeat bonuses of her sideways trajectory.

I felt weird about the conversation for hours afterward. Off. Wrong. But convinced myself I'd merely been trying to cheer her up.

Then the universe curve-balled me (puckish universe) the same situation in reverse. I was telling a friend how gutted I was about a fledgling relationship's demise, and she sunny-side-upped me, aggressively.

I found myself saying, 'But surely I'm allowed to feel a little disappointed, at least for a few days?' I felt like she'd invalidated my feelings, like I wasn't permitted. My emotions were not sanctioned.

And with that, I realized that I'd been the perky, non-empathic goat to my mate.

Sunny-side-upping can be great as an intervention when a friend is stuck in repetitive victim thinking, but I wonder if we're now going too far. After all, reams of research shows that suppressing negative emotions simply does not work. It's like trying not to think of a polar bear, and having a polar bear tap dance through your brain for the next hour.

It's abnormal to be happy all the time. 'Find ecstasy in life; the mere sense of living is joy enough,' Emily Dickinson once rhapsodized. I read this and felt immediately guilty that I'm not skipping around as if I'm in *The Sound of Music*. 'Ecstasy' is a bit strong love. Satisfaction would be more achievable.

It ticks us off even more, faking being happy when we're not. One study showed that those who work in public-facing jobs, who thus feel the pressure to be perpetually smiley, drink harder once they clock off from work.

The study's lead author, psychologist Alicia Grandey, was quoted as saying, 'The more they have to control negative emotions *at work*, the less they are able to control their alcohol intake *after work*'.

'Fake it until you make it' works with some things; confidence maybe. But with happiness, it does the exact opposite. Faking it makes us less happy. And horribly hungover the next day.

We're not supposed to be happy 24/7. It's spectacularly ordinary to feel sad occasionally.

The next time my mate tried to talk to me about her low mood due to her sideways career, I channelled the bear, listened and said, 'I'm sorry, I've felt like that too', and sat with her in the hole for a while holding her hand. That felt *right*.

ODES TO THE ORDINARY

An ode to garden-variety introverts

Laura: 'Where's D this weekend?'
Me: 'Taking some me-time.'
Laura: 'Mean-time?'
Me: 'Ha, no, ME-time.'

And then we spiralled off into how when we don't get me-time, it does become mean-time, because we need it to recharge before diving into the world again. Then we started saying we should make posters/mugs/ coasters with 'ME-TIME OR MEAN-TIME'.

I've needed a lot of me-time since I was a kid. Without it, I get depressed, ratty, snappy and can, if utterly deprived, become a right bitch. This is normal; because I'm an introvert. And introverts recharge by plugging into alone time. Without it, they flash red.

I know this about myself now, but it took me until age 33 to really figure this out. Before, I thought the solution to moods was to be with people, oh and to drink, as that's what popular culture had taught me.

I didn't know the solution was actually to be alone and not drink. Besides, I didn't really like being alone, back then, even though I needed it like oxygen. Because I didn't like myself, and this became all too evident when there was only myself in the room.

ODES TO THE ORDINARY
An ode to sunsets

We don't give the sky nearly enough credit. In the countryside, you'll see a ball of flame setting light to a gang of sulky, skinny trees on the horizon, while a plane blazes a cloud-comet-trail across the sky; a plane which holds hundreds of people currently eating a miniscule dinner.

Meanwhile, in our cities, sherbet powder bombs explode through the sky, above Regency beauties, on a clear night. On a cloudy night, the gloom and glow deepen until the clouds are backlit by neon. I mean.

And we pass it by. We don't stare slack-jawed at these nightly phenomena nearly often enough.

Not every night is spectacular, granted, but many are, and we mostly fail to stop and go 'holy shit' unless we are on holiday having a sundowner.

If the aliens are already here (check out the Jolie-Pitt kids – I have my suspicions they are intergalactic designer humans), they're losing their silvery minds over these sky showboats.

And we're just like – huh, ooh, OK *snap* – carries on.

Now, I stop, I look and I luxuriate in this free painting being created before my very eyes. Let's all give sunsets a little more credit, shall we, despite them being a nightly event.

'I'd shoot for the moon but I'm too busy gazing at stars.'

Eminem

ODES TO THE ORDINARY
An ode to never getting all your to-dos done

Did you know that only 59 per cent of to-do lists get ticked off each day? Yup. I would say with mine, given I have to-do eyes that are far larger than my belly, it's about 40 per cent.

I have three to-do lists on the go at any one time. A weekly one. A daily one, which normally consists of around 15 tasks. And a 'just do this' one, on which I write a single task at a time. To-do lists are largely considered by experts to be good; one study found that writing them before bed helps people fall asleep more quickly.

I sometimes rename my 'to do' as a 'want to do'. It reminds me of my own agency. Often the things you think you have to do, are actually things you want to do, says neuroscientist Dr Korb. 'The more you focus on the fact you *want to do it*, deep down, the more ultimately enjoyable it will be,' he explains.

But, there's a quirk to them. Once we've done something, once we've crossed it off, we instantly forget the task. We only remember what we *haven't* done.

We lie in bed, our brains abuzz with all the things we haven't done that day, feeling like an abject failure. The reality is, you've just forgotten the things you have done, says a psychological phenomenon called the Zeigarnik Effect. This was discovered by a Russian psychologist (Bluma Zeigarnik) while in a bustling restaurant in Vienna.

Zeigarnik realized that as soon as the waiters completed an order, they clean forgot about it. She then led studies that backed this up. 'We are more likely to remember and dwell on unfinished business than on completed tasks,' explains Professor Lyubomirsky

Now, I remember what I've done that day, rather than just what I haven't.

And when I start flipping out, I repeat these mantras:

I will never reach the end of my emails.
The house will never be 'done'.
The washing is an eternally propagating prophecy.

ORDINARY JOYS PART II

- Spraying a new suede/nubuck bag or shoes with protector, and feeling as if you have now given them a shield against The World.

- Having the newspaper delivered at the weekend.

- Doing a jubilant little jig after scoring a half-strike/strike in bowling.

- When a child brushes your hair with their fairy-soft touch.

- Leaping onto a train just as the doors are closing, and feeling a little like Liam Neeson (who recently said of those chucking him big bucks to do action flicks, 'Guys, I'm sixty-fucking-five').

- Learning basic phrases in Khmer, Polish or Welsh and getting a much friendlier reaction from locals, because most tourists don't bother their arse.

- Miniature things. Like travel toiletries. Dolls' house furniture. Model railway villages.

- Sending someone a letter rather than an email.

- Cracking an egg with one hand and feeling like a culinary school graduate.

- T-shirts that are genuinely funny. Today I saw a woman wearing 'Self-service only' and I wanted to fist-bump her.

- Alternative 'swears' around kids. 'Shut the front door!' or 'Oh, fudge'.

ODES TO THE ORDINARY
An ode to supremely lazy dinners

Sometimes, I'll leave the office at 8pm and stick two fingers up to the idea of cooking.

Instead, I spread some Doritos on a baking tray, smother them in jalapeños and grated cheese, melt, and serve with guacamole and sour cream.

I call this 'Nachos' to disguise the fact I am basically having crisps for dinner. I don't even plate them, I eat them directly out of the baking tray. It's disgusting and exquisite.

Other times, I'll have granola, yoghurt and banana, or beans on toast, or a fish finger sandwich – and it's heaven.

My friend Gemma is partial to putting cheese on crackers, serving it with olives and calling it a 'mezze'. Chloe is a fan of Weetabix with chocolate milk. My mate Ben has a Pot Noodle. (Names changed to protect the identities of the dirty diners.)

Now, I am not suggesting people eat this way all the time, because the nutritional value is basically nil, and if you do, you'll soon be able to roll yourself to the supermarket, like a beach ball with a face, for more chocolate milk and hash browns. But hell, it's nice to have a breather every now and then, and to eat like the kid from *Home Alone*, after a beast of a day.

I love my very ordinary, occasional workday dinners, and all the tabbouleh, or ceviche, or tagine in the world could not make me give them up. Let's hear it for the humble baked bean.

IV: ORDINARY LOVING

YOUR 'LOGICAL' FAMILY

I love that Armistead Maupin calls our friends our 'logical family', as a nod to the fact we have chosen them, whereas our 'biological family' are beyond our control.

I was not popular at school*. I wasn't socially excommunicated either, but I lived in the in-between land and was mostly ignored. So, I spent my twenties trying to redress that. I used to pride myself on how many picnic tables I could fill, basing my self-worth on how many jerk chicken dinners my birthday party ordered. I was labouring under the misconception that an extraordinary amount of friends was the ultimate. But I went for quantity over quality.

Thing is, it makes us unhappy to have too many close friends. Psychologists say it creates something called 'role strain'. Robin Dunbar, an evolutionary psychologist who has studied numbers of friends extensively, told the *Scientific American* that people ordinarily only have one or two 'special' buddies, plus five 'intimate' friends. These restricted numbers are reflected in more formal settings too, he says. 'For example, British Special Air Service squadrons have four men each.'

An extraordinary amount of close friends, even on a night out, is unmanageable. 'The limit of conversational laughter group size – say, at a bar – is about three people, which is slightly below the limit for conversation group size, which is four,' adds Dunbar. It follows that a dinner party for four people is going to be much more of a hit than one for ten.

I friend-edited rigorously in my mid-thirties, which I think is a fairly common time for a cull, asking myself the simple yet fiendishly effective question: 'Do I feel better or worse after I see them?' I then recently found myself in the market for more friends, having moved to a new city, and found that friend dating as an adult is peculiarly *more* nerve-frazzling than actual dating.

If they don't message you back after that 'do we like each other enough?' coffee, it's not as if you can tell yourself a reassuring bedtime story that they got back with an ex, or met someone else, or maybe they're 'not ready' to commit to the festival of sexiness that is you. The only story is: they just didn't want to hang out with you again. But, that's OK. Nobody gets every friend they're grooming.

---

* I am grateful for that in retrospect, having watched how the 'populars' lives have played out on Facebook. Spells in prison have featured.

It's undeniable though, that a small, carefully chosen 'logical family' gives our life meaning. There was a famous research project, The Grant Study, which followed every aspect of the lives of 268 men for three decades. The study threw up many interesting findings, one of which was that drinking was the most significant cause of divorce. But the most important discovery, said the study's leader George Vaillant, was this one. 'The only thing that really matters in life are your relationships to other people.' Whether romantic or platonic.

I'll leave you with this remarkable finding. In her book *The Myths of Happiness*, Professor Lyubomirsky cites a study in which researchers asked participants to look at a hill and later describe how steep it was. 'Incredibly, those who were accompanied by a friend – especially a friend they were close to and knew a long time – judged the hill to be *less steep* than those who were alone,' she says.

Turns out a friend can literally help you see a mountain as more of a molehill.

SHRINKING OUR SKYSCRAPER-TALL EXPECTATIONS OF RELATIONSHIPS

'So we come to one person, and we basically are asking them
to give us what once an entire village used to provide: Give
me belonging, give me identity, give me continuity, but
give me transcendence and mystery and awe all in one. Give
me comfort, give me edge. Give me novelty, give me
familiarity. Give me predictability, give me surprise. And we
think it's a given, and toys and lingerie are going to save us
with that.'

Esther Perel, psychotherapist

This Esther Perel quote is *everything*. It so neatly sums up the contradictions
we seek in our romantic relationships. From our partners, we expect what
was once provided to us by an entire village. Security and spontaneity,
predictability and wildness, the soft and the sharp. We look to them for things
that cannot co-exist.

Feel free to hold out for a relationship that feels extraordinary at the get-
go. I'm a fan of that. But bear in mind that no matter how 'extra' it is in the
beginning, it will always, always hedonically adapt until it feels ordinary.

Here are some unavoidable truths:

- In the beginning, you're so hyper-aware of their proximity to you, that
it's as exhilarating as a safari lion padding into your personal space. Yet,
this inexorably mellows until it's more tiger...then more cheetah...and
eventually, akin to a house cat. They become smaller, less glamorous and
less dangerous over time and there's jack shit we can do about it.

- When you first touch your partner you feel that 'bjjjjjhhhhh' taser jolt of lust,
yet once you've touched them 500 times, it downgrades to a mere flicker.

- When you first see them nude, it's like you've just clapped eyes on Michelangelo's *David* – or Praxiteles's *Aphrodite* – while two years in, their naked body is as commonplace as the washing machine.

- The first time you hear them whistle tunelessly it's adorable; once you live together it drives you bananas.

It's just the inevitable science of adaptation. Turning what feels extraordinary at first, into the ordinary. Your irritation or indifference is not a thought-crime. What's important to realize, is that even if we were dating Chris Hemsworth or Mila Kunis, the exact same process would occur.

It's like how – once things are on our Netflix 'watchlists' they gradually drain of any appeal, until we no longer want to 'watch' them. It's like how – the longer we own a book, the less we want to read it, even though we were hot for it upon point of purchase. They are netted butterflies, that lose allure the longer we own them, so we bound out to search for more.

It's up to us to know about this illusion, so that we can outwit it.

Our disposability mindset

Hilda Burke, an integrative psychotherapist and couples counsellor, believes that our disappointed expectations are a result of not only hedonic adaptation, but also shifting cultural sands. 'For our grandparents, marriage truly was for life; divorces were very rare.'

And divorces were stigmatized, even when they did become possible. Burke raises the example of Ireland, where divorce was outlawed until 1995 and, even then, it only got approved by an edge of 0.28 per cent that voted 'for' in the referendum.

When asked about his five decades' strong marriage to my grandma, my Irish grandfather used to joke, 'Why would I want another woman? I've been working on this one *for ages* and she's almost perfect.'

Obviously divorce is still a huge, life-altering decision, but when you're just dating, Burke likens the disposability mindset we now have around clothes to how we see modern relationships. 'No one mends clothes anymore, not really; we just chuck them and buy new ones. I wonder if this mentality is feeding into relationships too.' My grandparents darned socks; now, we wouldn't dream of it.

Given there are thousands upon thousands of people sitting in an app, waiting for us to 'heart' them, Burke says it's now harder to see things through. 'What if there's someone out there that I match better with?' The unopened doors, untried partners haunt us and tempt us.

'The paradox is that too much choice makes it more difficult to choose,' says Burke. 'We keep trying, trying, trying, until we find the "perfect person". Only problem is, the "perfect person" is a myth.' A myth that we chase to our detriment.

What's more, monogamy as a social construct was invented when we were only likely to live around half as long as we do now. 'If you get married at 30,' says Burke 'and you both live until say 90, which now is very much possible, you are looking at 60 years of fidelity. Some would argue that monogamy is not necessarily designed to last as long as we do now.' A strong argument for later marriages, if only we could silence those deafening biological clocks (which tyrannize all genders; for the record, the tick-tock is not the reserve of females).

Erecting the expectations

I once heard the phrase 'expectations are resentments under construction' in a recovery meeting. It triggered a silent revolution in my brain. By expecting so much from people, I was actually setting myself up for disappointment.

Romcoms play a huge part, particularly if you're female, in constructing these lofty expectations, intensifying the urge to jettison things that are less than perfect.

Take a romcom I recently saw – *Modern Life is Rubbish*. Major spoilers ahead. This is a lovely, quirky movie (in which Blur are depicted as a vintage band, which is mildly terrifying). But its depiction of a twenty-tens romance is outlandishly unrealistic.

The main female character turns down a trip to Florence with Eligible Bloke A, because Eligible Bloke B (her ex) just went viral with a love song that's indubitably about her.

Meanwhile, Bloke B is totally destroyed by the break-up, can't eat or sleep, and winds up having a mild breakdown on stage.

So, Bloke B sends her a box o' stuff that would have taken him about a week to make and arrange; an iPhone with a playlist, a treasure hunt of clues and tickets around London via boat, rickshaw and cable car. Then, random people hand her flowers, a suitcase and a retro photo viewer, until the crescendo of the finale; a picnic proposal.

Here's the thing. I don't know anyone who's ever found themselves with two people in love with them simultaneously, both of whom they could opt for. No one! I've had handmade cards and flowers and picnics before, but never all simultaneously. I've had romantic partners apologize and ask for me back before, but the delivery of the 'I was a plonker, please forgive me' is usually just a text or at most, a phone call.

From the male point of view, this narrative, and many others besides, tells them that unless *they can't live without the person*, unless they feel inspired to pen songs about them, it's probably not worth pursuing. Equally, I don't know any men who have experienced this.

I used to constantly expect these levels of romanticism, I used to say 'I just want you to fight for me' a lot, but given I don't do any of the above either, why should I expect it from them?

Behold the extraordinary couple on socials

We are living in an age of many, many ultra-visible couples on social media. They do ironic Christmas cards of them with their dog. They brag about the 'best boyfriend everrr' bringing them breakfast in bed; or he captions a picture of her laughing with 'She's the best'. They look good in a restaurant, in a glass lift, with their heads on the pillow.

But hold up, why are they taking pictures of themselves in bed? Surely if you're in bed with someone and you want to take pictures, rather than spoon, or indeed, fork, then something is amiss?

A 2014 study of more than 100 couples cheekily entitled 'Can you tell I'm in a relationship?' found that there's a strong link between insecurity and frequent social media posting. 'When people felt more insecure about their partner's feelings, they tended to make their relationships visible,' the paper's authors wrote. It seems Barbie and Ken doth protest too much.

'I've seen a lot of couples kissing on social media of late, and not just a peck; deeply kissing,' says couples counsellor Hilda Burke. 'If it's not a selfie, I often think, "who's the person taking this picture?" Either way, what appears to be intimate, is actually very choreographed.'

She says that if you need confirmation online about the value of your relationship, it's often like the person who puts a swimwear photo up to garner praise. 'The very posting of the picture can often mean there's an insecurity there – that the person posting is trying to resolve.'

The honeymoon dismantled

The honeymoon period is elevated as that extraordinary time when your senses are sharpened, as if you're a newborn vampire; you can see no wrong in your partner, only right; and when everything has a pink, fuzzy filter laid over it. It is also traditionally meant to be the time when you do things like row boats together, try on comedy glasses in joke shops, or do bad karaoke.

But what if it's a time of more strife, than euphoria? What if the start is more ordinary, than extraordinary? Or if it's actually stressful? Personally, I find the beginning of a relationship petrifying. That low rumble of incoming love is unsettling to me; like an oncoming train when I'm bound to the tracks. Intoxicating and exhilarating too, but mostly just scary. It's once things settle down, say six months on, once I know they're not going to ghost me, or cheat, or do a midnight flit after sex, that I start to breathe and really enjoy it.

The honeymoon is also not necessarily when things are rose-scented and perfect. 'If things aren't great now, when you're in the honeymoon period, what are they going to be like six years down the line?!' is a frequently wheeled-out social belief system. All the while, these people are conveniently ignoring the bumps they experienced at the start. The ex they wanted back instead, the time they dumped them for acting like a knucklehead, the early-on infidelity.

They would never say that about the first six months at a job, when they know you'll be settling in, ironing out kinks, figuring out what to do/not to do. They would never say that about parenting, or driving, or wakeboarding, or a friendship, or any new activity/person that we have to get used to.

We know that starts are bumpy, in all other realms of existence. So why do we apply that 'if it's not perfect, torpedo it' pink-cloud pressure to newborn relationships, which are already wobbly-legged? I think the 'honeymoon period' expectation sticks its leg out and trips up many relationships before they've even gotten into their stride.

'There is a societal collusion around perpetuating honeymoon expectations,' agrees Hilda Burke. And not everyone enjoys the first stage, she says; what is one person's elixir, is another's poison. 'It depends a lot on your attachment style*. Those with an insecure attachment pattern find the uncertainty of it intensely anxiety-provoking, and are prone to nix things prematurely as a result.'

---

* If you don't know what we're on about, and you're curious, try searching online for 'attachment style quiz' and a host of options will pop up for you to figure out where you sit on the spectrum.

Whereas those who are sitting pretty in a secure attachment style, can absolutely love it. 'They feel safe on the "will we, won't we become official" ride,' Burke says. New partners are also a blank canvas, she says, which means we can sketch in fantasies of who they might be. 'We don't know them very well, so the opportunities for projection are massive. They can still be everything we want them to be. We haven't met their difficult mother yet, and they haven't seen what we're like when we're hangry.'

This 'best side' phase is unsustainable, because frankly, it's exhausting. 'The grooming routine in particular,' laughs Burke. 'We're keeping our faces, bodies and the undesirable parts of our personality in check.'

It's seen as a charmed chapter, but the honeymoon is more aptly described as a phase of pretence. Fantasy, before reality sets in. And 'reality' comes with benefits. We can stop analysing their facial expressions, or second-guessing what that behaviour meant, and start to star-shape into the security.

The 'honeymoon period' is hugely over-rated. And often, a lot bumpier than we're led to anticipate.

When you say tomato and they say tomayto

One of the most discombobulating, mystifying things about relationships, is how you can remember the exact same event in totally different ways, or how one of you can remember a conversation with word-for-word, pin-perfect accuracy, while the other thinks it never happened. But, this too, is incredibly ordinary.

Once you excavate the science behind it, it becomes clear as to why this continually happens. We think of our memories as facts. As faithfully recorded episodes, mental videos, word-for-word transcriptions of our personal history.

The reality is, if your memory files are books in a library, they are books that have been written by someone highly biased (yourself). On top of that, every time you retrieve them from the shelves paragraphs get redacted, notes get scribbled in the margins and words are highlighted.

It's overwhelmingly been proven that if you interview a bunch of witnesses just after an event, they'll mostly report the same sequence of events. The longer you leave it, the more disparate the memories become. Time is a great memory-distorter.

Hilda Burke, who has worked with hundreds of couples as a counsellor, says that she sees this all the time. 'Even to the level where one says the argument happened on Monday night, while the other swears blind it was

Tuesday. One thinks it was in the kitchen, the other the living room.'

Neither are lying, she says, it's just that our memories become distorted and patchy. 'Our memories of arguments are not just filtered; they're triple-filtered. By your confirmation bias (which seeks to back up your view of the world), how you view yourself, and how you view your partner.' The result is that you feed the same argument into two brains, and two completely different stories churn out.

Professor Lyubomirsky says one of her favourite studies shows that couples experience altogether 'different realities'. A 1981 study took dozens of couples and asked each partner about the events of the past week; had they fought, had sex, watched TV, resolved a problem with the kids? 'The amazing finding from this study is that husbands and wives completely failed to agree with each other,' she says.

So, your memory contradictions are not unusual. They're maddening, yet to be expected.

The dance of relationships

It's tremendously normal for a coupleship to look a lot like a aerially-viewed dance. In the beginning, it's often a clumsy shitshow. Sometimes one moves more towards the other; sometimes one bounces away; sometimes one falls; sometimes you both move in perfect unison.

Let's look to an unlikely hero for this: Gwyneth Paltrow's father. 'I asked my dad once, "How did you and Mum stay married for 33 years?", Gwyneth told *Glamour* magazine in 2013. 'And he said, "Well, we never wanted to get divorced at the same time."'

'It's normal for one person in a couple to hold down the fort, if the other is having a hard time and doesn't have the mental bandwidth to be loving,' says Hilda Burke.

One picks up the slack and keeps things chugging along. 'That's healthy give-and-take. But a more extreme pursuer-avoidant dynamic can be a dysfunctional seesaw. If one comes forward, the other steps back. It means there's always a safe distance between them, and true intimacy is never established.'

Taking advice with a pinch of salt

It can be incredibly confusing, says Hilda Burke, to receive altogether conflicting advice. And there is no such thing as objective advice from a friend or family member. 'As the author Anais Nin says, "We don't see things as they are, we see them as *we* are."'

'When we're single, we tend to want our friends to match us,' says Burke, 'whereas when we're in a couple, we want a pair to double date with. This validates our own choices. Also, everyone has different needs, codes and values, meaning what might be unthinkable for your friend, is no big deal for you.'

I really relate to this advice bias. There have definitely been times in the past when I have advised friends to 'knock it on the head' because I was single and wanted them to be single too, even though my bias was unconscious.

'Also, your friends are naturally inclined to want to stick up for you, to sympathize with you,' says Burke. Materializing in outrage of the 'Did he/she really say that to you?!' ilk. But, you're giving them a skewed version of events, they are not hearing your partner's story, and they don't get the context either. They only get the hurtful missile he/she/they lobbed. 'It's the equivalent of zeroing in on what's in the foreground, and ignoring the background of day-to-day good stuff,' points out Burke.

Here's the thing. Nobody knows whether a relationship is worth pursuing, saving, or resurrecting, other than the two people in it. We don't phone our friends and family about the serene weekend we just had that featured one of us rubbing the other's back for an hour at 2am because of glamorous trapped wind. We don't give blow-by-blow 'then he said, then I said' accounts of fun conversations. We don't tell them in great detail about them teaching us to play tennis, or the roast they made, or the apricot Vans he/she thoughtfully bought for you.

We tend to only tell them about the extra-bad stuff, like the yelled argument, or the extraordinary stuff, such as the gorgeous holiday. If our relationships were skyscrapers, our family and friends only get to see the first two floors (the hellish) and the penthouse (the heavenly). There are ten floors of ordinary, everyday, unremarkable getting-on that they just don't see.

Extraordinary relationships are a myth

Belgian psychotherapist Esther Perel is now my North Star when it comes to relationship navigation. She helps me remember that eternally extraordinary relationships are about as real as unicorns that fart glitter.

She wrote a book called *Mating in Captivity*; a clever titled nod to the ennui – or bored pacing – that sets in once we're caged in long-term relationships. The irreconcilable tussle between social norm and evolutionary hardwiring.

We're told the ideal is to marry for life, and yet we're not programmed for that, so the result is akin to a couple of giant pandas who refuse to do it, despite prods from the zookeepers, a breathlessly awaiting public and piped-in Barry White warbling.

Here are my favourite Perel quotes. I need to print them onto the insides of my eyelids, since I forget them constantly. Drifting accidentally into the infested waters of idealism once more, where the sharks of my own expectations glide noiselessly beneath the surface, waiting to take me and my latest relationship down.

- '[Love is] a verb....It's an active engagement with all kinds of feelings. Positive ones and primitive ones and loathsome ones. But it's a very active verb. And it's often surprising how it can kind of ebb and flow. It's like the moon. We think it's disappeared, and suddenly it shows up again. It's not a permanent state of enthusiasm.'

You may well disagree, given our belief system around 'what love is' tends to be a very complicated cascade of nurture and experiences, but somewhere along the way I picked up the (in retrospect, juvenile) notion that love is supposed to be a constant, that *just happens* to a person, like we catch the common cold, independent of effort or activity. Yeah. Maybe not.

- 'It's natural that people argue. Its part of intimacy. But you have to have a good system of repair. You need to be able to go back, if you've lost it, which happens, and say "I brought in my dirty tricks, I'm sorry", or "You know what, I realized I didn't hear a single word you said because I was so upset, can we talk about it again?"'

When arguments do happen, I am so conflict-shy now that I have an itchy trigger finger for the ruby-red 'Eject Passenger' button. I am prone to being so uncomfortable with a confrontation, that I attempt to avoid it by simply removing the person from my life. Which is obviously far from ideal, given arguments are ordinary and to be expected. Maybe you relate?

- '[Cheating] isn't so much that they want to leave the person that they are with, sometimes they want to leave the person that they have *themselves* become.'

Back when I was addicted to alcohol, I cheated on partners I loved deeply, which was absolutely nothing to do with them; and everything to do with me being trapped in the seventh circle of hell that is active addiction.

Being blackout drunk wrestles all control from our rational selves and gives the steering wheel to what amounts to a monkey driving a car. During a blackout, the hippocampus stops creating new memories. I wasn't trying to escape my partner, I was trying to escape myself via wine, so much so that infidelities were the horrifying result.

Ever since I quit drinking in 2013, my fidelity record has been flawless, which is no coincidence. If your pattern is also 'drink 'n' cheat', I highly recommend removing the 'drink' and seeing if the 'cheat' vanishes too... surprisingly effortlessly.

Escalator relationships

I think it has to be said in the overarching theme of embracing your 'ordinary relationship' that moving in together, although it can be lovely, is also incredibly hard work.

Pockmarked with pitfalls and fraught with speedbumps that slow your former lust to a crawl. Less sex, more squabbling about why the other thinks it's OK to not wipe down the kitchen. Less talking, more unspoken resentments elbowing each other in the silence.

And as soon as you move in together, here's what happens next. People start asking when you're going to get married. The 'escalator relationship' that is endorsed by society means that you get nagged and badgered into the next phase, even if you have no desire to go there just yet, or ever.

Intriguingly, I've been told by two gay friends of mine that now that same-sex marriage is legal, they are being stalked by the same societal 'escalator expectations'. 'We felt pretty free of that before,' one told me. 'The most we could do was live together, or have/adopt a baby. But now it's all, "when are you getting married?" We're suddenly on the same escalator as straight couples, and many of us are not enjoying that extra pressure,' she said, empathetically.

The best piece of advice I've ever received about 'ordinary' relationships, was this belter. 'Lower your expectations of people, and up your gratitude, and you'll find your relationships improve immeasurably.' It altered my very foundations, like a subtle seismic shift which alters continental plates irrevocably.

Grasping for that heart-shaped balloon never made me happy, anyway. It just made me...grasping.

IN PURSUIT OF THE SEX-TRAORDINARY

I worked at *Cosmopolitan* magazine in my mid-twenties, including a very brief spell as 'Sex Editor'. As part of my job, I had to do things like hit the street and find women who were willing to be named, pictured and to answer the question, 'How does it feel when you have your G-spot stimulated?'

I was in charge of our 'penis reader' column, featuring a batshit crazy lady who thought she could read a penis like a palm. This meant she needed pictures of real penises. I had to send texts to my friends saying, 'I know this sounds really pervy, but if I send you a disposable camera, could you please take some pictures of Rob's ding-dong for this "penis reader" column thing?'

Follow up text: 'PS. Oh and could you also provide a pic of you as a couple, so that we can print that. OK, thanksbyeeee'.

I mean, what?! A number of my friends did it too.

Given I was writing and editing all of these wackadoodle tips such as using an unexpected ice cube during oral sex, smothering yourself in whipped cream, and surprising him with a lap dance, I ended up thinking that missionary was a total cop-out, and sex wasn't good unless it resembled something porn-like, unless I'd ticked off five positions within 20 minutes.

This led to some questionable decisions on my part in an attempt to reach an erotic wonderland. 'It doesn't have to be this complicated,' a few sexual partners said to me, as I was throwing myself around.

You may be surprised to learn how often people are actually having sex, as opposed to what they tell you. Data on over 26,000 American couples showed that the average pair has sex once a week. And surprisingly, upturning a common urban myth, married couples only had sex on average three times less a year compared to the unmarried (51 times, as opposed to 54).

The notion that older people have less sex is also a fallacy. 'Age is not as important a factor as people think,' says Professor Lyubomirsky. 'If you want to predict how often a couple engages in sex, you'd be much more accurate if you considered how long they'd been together, rather than their age.'

The secure sex swan dive

I've been in many fledgling relationships where, after a demure courtship dance, we will tumble into bed and have sex...I dunno...five times in 24 hours. I don't even know I'm doing it; my body just tells me to.

But what was I actually doing? Very likely this: trying to bed him into wanting to commit to me. Shag to snag. Which has backfired a number of times, when I've then been placed into the 'fun times only' box, and thus have accidentally shagged my way out of ever being introduced to his mother.

Once I feel secure in a relationship, my libido takes a swan dive. Three times a week is plenty...two even. And I think this happens a lot.

'The sex drive naturally wanes across both genders in long-term relationships,' says Professor Lyubomirsky. But contrary to the societal assumption that men lose interest faster, 'the adaptation is actually faster for women'. Women are more novelty-seeking than men, she says.

The reality is this. I now know that all you have to do to have good sex is show up, make sure you're washed, say things like 'what do you like?', concentrate on pleasure rather than pain (unless pain is your bag) and...that's it. Ordinary sex is good sex.

A BUDGET WEDDING AND WHY IT MEANS YOU'RE LESS LIKELY TO DIVORCE

We're told that extraordinary weddings are supersized demonstrations of commitment. And yet, the truth is the exact opposite. The more ordinary the better. Data shows that the more you spend on your wedding, the more likely you are to divorce. Yes, really.

In the brilliantly titled 2014 paper, '"A Diamond is Forever" and Other Fairy Tales', two top economists looked at 3,000 American couples and discovered that it's a big frothy myth that an extravagant wedding is an omen for long-lasting marital bliss. 'The wedding industry has consistently sought to link wedding spending with long-lasting marriages,' they wrote. 'We found that marriage duration is either not associated or inversely associated with spending on the engagement ring and wedding ceremony.'

Specifically, they discovered that spending less than $1,000 on the wedding day meant the 'hazard of divorce' was half as likely, while spending $20,000 or more led to an inflation of that risk to the power of 1.6. Sheesh.

I wonder if Kristen Bell and Dax Shepard knew this when, despite having a combined net worth of many millions, they decided to have a $142 wedding at a courthouse.

This report also melted down the perception that men who spend a month's salary on an engagement ring are more committed. A $2,000 to $4,000 engagement ring was associated with a 1.3 times greater hazard of divorce, when compared to rings that cost between $500 and $2,000.

Another fascinating thing the study threw up was that marrying for superficial reasons shortens the marriage's shelf-life. 'Reporting that one's partner's looks were important in the decision to marry is significantly associated with shorter marriage duration,' Professor Hugo Mialon, one of the study's authors, told *The Independent*.

Even though a honeymoon adds more to the overall bill, the same report showed that 'having a honeymoon is associated with a lower hazard of divorce'. It didn't matter if it was a budget weekend, it seems, since they add, 'regardless of how much the honeymoon cost'. So, even a few days in a campervan counts.

Wedding vows for those who know wedding rings are not magical jewellery that bestow eternal conjugal bliss upon the wearer

Do I get a prize for the longest subtitle ever? No?

There's a brilliant trend in recent times to jettison the 'til death do us part' line of the vows, sending it into a room of redundant antiquated knick-knacks, along with the promise to 'obey'.

Modern brides and grooms are choosing instead to opt for much more realistic vows, such as 'For as long as we continue to love each other', 'For as long as our love shall last' and 'Until our time together is over'.

These reflect the increasing acknowledgement that an ended marriage is not necessarily a 'failed' one, given the many happy years together. Brad Pitt tore up the rule book by refusing to label his ended marriage to Jennifer Aniston as a 'failure', instead telling *W* magazine that he saw it 'as a total success...that's five more [years] than I made it with anyone else'.

Similarly, Jennifer Aniston is singing from the same happily divorced hymn sheet. 'My marriages, they've been very successful, in (my) personal opinion,' she told *Elle* magazine of her five-year union with Brad Pitt and her two-and-a-half year marriage to Justin Theroux. 'And when they came to an end,' said Jennifer, 'it was a choice that was made because we chose to be happy, and sometimes happiness didn't exist within that arrangement anymore'.

If I ever get married, these will be my vows.

I can live without you but I choose not to.

This is not unconditional love, it is deep love with healthy boundaries.

This is not a happy ever after, it is the beginning of our biggest challenge as a couple.

You are not my everything; but you are one of my favourite things.

I have no idea if this will last forever, given I am not a prophet, but I hope it does.

You do not complete me, given only I can do that, but I feel like you mostly bring forth the best parts of me.

This is not perfect, but then, nothing is.

I cannot wait to spend an as-yet-undefined, yet no doubt significant portion of my life with you.

I enter this with clear eyes, an open heart and my sleeves rolled up.

BREAK-UPS ARE MORE COMMON THAN NOT

Most relationships break up. And even if the twosome defies all odds and makes it to marriage, over four in ten couples then tumble into being a divorce statistic. Most relationships are not built to last.

I've said this before, but our society tends to go 'Oh well, *that* didn't work then' when a relationship ends. But just because it ended, it doesn't mean it wasn't wondrous.

Here's a diary entry I wrote not so long ago about a relationship.

We are very different. Maybe too different. This has not been conflict free.

He is the kind of person who scrunches recipes up and freestyles, who sets fire to Ikea assembly instructions while cackling, while that kind of caper makes my instruction-following blood run cold. He says 'why do today what you can do tomorrow', which makes my eyeball twitch.

He is spiritual while I am an unapologetic atheist who gives any attempts to 'open my mind to spirituality' short shrift, and once threatened to go to beatnik-mecca Ubud in Bali, wearing a T-shirt saying, 'Crystals are just pretty rocks'.

Speaking of crystals, last week he had a strained groin. I suggested he put a hot water bottle on it, and he replied, 'Nah, I've got a crystal on there that was blessed by the Dalai Lama.' I'm recording all of these lines to send to Sacha Baron Cohen for a future character.

I like to work, listen to music, clean, watch TV, read or exercise the entire time I'm awake, while he appears to spend a lot of time 'in stillness', which I find utterly confounding.

I believe that good things happen because you work freaking hard for them, while he manifests things by calling upon Gaia (a Greek goddess) while I try really hard not to chuckle and roll my non-believing eyes. And then I sit back, puzzled, as his way appears to work just as well as mine.

It's like he lives under a rock. Once I asked him if he wanted to get a Deliveroo. 'What's that?' he replied. 'I know what a kangaroo is, but what's a Deliveroo?' And then there was the time I mentioned someone was a 'Millennial'.

'What's a Millennial?' he asked, baffled.
'Are you shitting me?' I said.
'No,' he replied. 'Are they something to do with the Millennium Falcon?'

To this day, even though he now knows what they are, he calls them 'millenniums'.

He calls me Polly, because I'm always putting the kettle on. He lives in the middle of noplace where everybody knows each other's name, and his home is lit exclusively by Himalayan salt rock lamps that throw rosy shadows against six foot scores of driftwood. He says things like, 'I wonder if we know them?' when a tracing-paper butterfly follows us down the street, and he has a half-feral, jet-black cat who burnishes auburn under the summer sun.

He has seven guitars that he etches art on and gives away freely when he meets someone special who could do with a guitar but can't afford one. When people ask how old he is, he sometimes says 'timeless' with an impish smile on his face, but he half means it. He calls London 'The Death Star' and is anarchistic to his bones, and yet was captain of the cricket team at school.

We curve around each other like speech marks around things yet unsaid. Skate-park bashed copper against Irish cream. Inked on his skin are geckos, a ghoul wearing an Indiana Jones hat and poetry about it not being the destination, but the glory of the ride, while mine is a cowardly middle-class blank canvas, aside from an imperceptible dot where I once had my nose pierced in the hope it would make me a rebel, only for my mum to say it was 'cool' and my dad to jovially ask when I was planning on running away and joining The Breeders.

In many ways, we're a walking contradiction of a couple. I once had a pair of iron figurines that were either vigorously opposed to one another, or passionately magnetized, depending on which way you flipped them; and that is how we are.

Our clashes may end up breaking us. We may stop spending the majority of our time in 'passionately magnetized' and end up spending most of it in 'vigorously opposed'.

Our relationship is like living in an electric thunderstorm. It's exquisite and devastating. I don't know if I can live in a thunderstorm long-term.

Turns out I couldn't. That relationship did end. But that doesn't mean it wasn't a force of nature, and a marvel that I'm eternally grateful to have experienced.

When it's underordinary

But generally, relationships break up because it's not extraordinary or ordinary; it's underordinary (yep, just made that word up). There's a distinction between 'ordinary' fighting and the systematic destruction of each other's self-esteem. An 'ordinary' lull and the rising damp of indifference. An 'ordinary' sex drought and an arid desert.

It's been shown that we need five positive experiences, within a relationship, to every negative experience – in order to keep it 'happy'. Why? As we now know, our brains give the negatives precedence; they are bigger, badder and stronger in our heads. The interplay between negative and positive within a relationship is like a WWF wrestler having a tug of war against a ten-year-old kid. (It's a hard knock life, kid. You're not gonna win. Perhaps go and get four of your buddies and you *might*.)

So, given the five-to-one golden rule, if the negatives multiply and the positives diminish, you will find yourself at that dispiriting crossroads of 'STAY' and 'LEAVE'. The crossroads of continue and get to keep them, but potentially lose yourself. Or let go, and endure the pain of losing them, but keep yourself.

You stand there for weeks, months, years, confounded. Paralysed by the fear of what people will say, what you will do, who you will be without them.

Until you take a deep breath, sling your bundled wherewithal over your shoulder on a stick, and set off down the 'LEAVE' path.

But the first portion of the 'LEAVE' path is an enchanted Tim Burton-esque path, wicked with self-doubt and reality-bending. It tries to get you to turn back.

You can no longer hear the pin-bright coalmine canary you must have heard dozens, hundreds of times, pealing the alarm of toxicity. Instead, whispers press up against you saying, 'What have you done?', or 'Love conquers all, doesn't it?', and 'Was it really that bad? I don't think so!' or 'Now you will be alone forever, y'know'.

That slideshow of bad times that whirred through your mind is whipped away, and a trailer of good times is inserted. You start to think you've made the worst decision of your existence thus far.

But the canary was real. If it hadn't been, what you were you doing at the crossroads in the first place? Why did you spend all of that time staring at the 'LEAVE' and 'STAY' arrows? The you that stood at the crossroads for a heckofalong time chose this path for good bloody reason.

You forge on.

And then, just as you think the 'LEAVE' path harpies have given up and gone to fuck with someone else's grip on reality, you will reach into a parrot-bright summer bag and find your hand around sun lotion that makes you whimper with loss, given the last time you wore it, you two were happy and intact.

The animal-trap pain from closing your hand around an everyday item; the teleportation induced by a song; the ability for a smell on an item of clothing to tip you onto the floor. It's a form of bereavement. And no great wonder, given the person you shared a bed, baths, cars, hammocks and dreams with has suddenly been shorn from your life. Snip.

If you were the one who did the leaving, there's this sensation. Conviction and self-doubt elbowing each other in your head for dominance. This is typical of 'cognitive dissonance', the stressful push-pull of a dilemma, of making/having made any significant relationship decision.

The only way to calm your brain down, says neuroscience, is to hold fast to and trust the decision. To constantly say, 'brain, thanks for that, but I am resolute'.

And if you were the one who was left, your mind promptly erases all the times you had doubts too, so hellbent is it on distressing the injury of having been left. And so you repeat that this break-up was for the best, for the best, forthebest. That they simply did what you were not strong enough to. That you're glad that you now know that they're indifferent, that they don't see a future, or that they were shagging their ex, Sarah.

Eventually, finally, at long last, the psychological torture eases, your brain starts falling in with the approved script you keep repeating at it, the one created by your 'higher brain', and peace is finally yours.

It's like the end of the world, and the beginning of it, all smushed up into one. Like you'll go insane from the back-and-forth, but you don't. Like the canaries weren't real, even though you know they were.

It's devastating, yet strangely intoxicating, because hot damn do you feel like an exposed electric wire of grief and possibilities right now. Now you can rediscover who you are, what you want, who you *can* be. Like every negative, break-ups have a faint glow of positive, if you look really, really hard.

Putting all your future happiness in their hands

I now know that my reaction to a break-up has always depended heavily on how much power I have given the relationship over my perceived future happiness.

When the break-up has abso-fricking-lutely decimated me, it has done so for one reason; I made the romantic relationship, and the survival of it, the centre of my existence. All my hope was based on it working out. So, when it ended, my hope was utterly eclipsed and my life plunged into darkness. Funtimes!

Here's a handy diagram of that eclipse...

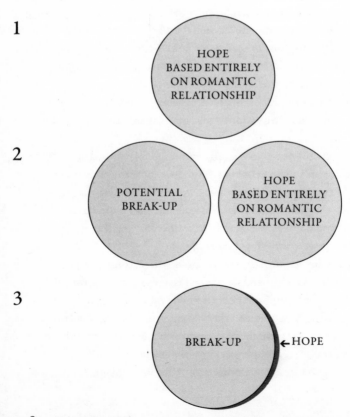

1

HOPE
BASED ENTIRELY
ON ROMANTIC
RELATIONSHIP

2

POTENTIAL
BREAK-UP

HOPE
BASED ENTIRELY
ON ROMANTIC
RELATIONSHIP

3

BREAK-UP ← HOPE

Even when I am seeing someone now, I always have my hopeful single future firmly in mind too; writing more books, an indecent amount of travelling, and hopefully a farmhouse, a horse called Jimi Hendrix, a goose called Cher and ducklings called Bros.

I know now that I can be just as happy single as I am in a relationship. Which is the kind of statement die-hard 'romantic love is everything!' believers would find to be anathema. 'Well, you shouldn't be with them then!' they would cry. I feel like Richard Curtis would stamp on this statement, if I laid it at his starry-eyed feet.

And yet it's true. Because as much as relationships are lovely, they are also chuffing challenging, and the loveliness and the challenge balance out to make it much the same, for me.

If you're single, pinning your hope and imagined future on whatever-new paramour is a dangerous gamble. Whereas, architecting a happy single future even if *nothing ever works out* is a sure bet.

And for those of you in solid, happy relationships, daring to construct an alternative mental image of a single future that *is also happy*, can provide you with a psychological escape chute should things falter. It means you don't feel as if you've painted yourself into a corner.

What's your alternative, happy single future?

THE MYTH THAT SINGLE IS AN UNDERORDINARY EXISTENCE

There's an absurd meme doing the rounds right now: 'One day somebody will hug you so hard all your broken pieces will stick back together'. Awww NOPE.

Nobody has the power to do that, unless they're a Marvel character bestowed with some sort of mental health superglue. The heavy lifting on happiness is all down to us. Being in a couple, or getting hitched, does not inoculate you from being unhappy, at all.

In fact, it's well known among psychologists that marriage only provides a brief vault in happiness. 'Research shows convincingly that married people are no happier than single ones,' says Professor Lyubomirsky. She cites an investigation that tracked 1,761 people who got married and stayed married over 15 years.

'This study found that newlyweds derive a happiness boost from getting married that lasts an average of about two years.' Professor Lyubomirsky goes onto say that while married women spend more time having sex and less time alone than their single counterparts; they also spend less time with friends, reading or watching TV.

But, the Marriage Superiority Committee really don't like hearing about findings such as this. Recently, a piece about Paul Dolan's work went viral, which was entitled 'Women are happier without a child or a spouse, says happiness expert', and appeared in the *Guardian*. And boy, did this put the proverbial cat among the pigeons. The reaction from married people was, in Paul Dolan's own words, 'furious' and 'revealed the strength of "married is best" prejudice'.

Meanwhile, Revolut hit the press for single-shaming, with headlines like 'Backlash over "single shaming" banking ad' (*BBC News*). They put out an ad saying, 'To the 12,750 people who ordered a single takeaway on Valentine's Day. You OK, hun?' Which has apparently nothing to do with banking, other than making their single customers feel as if they're spying on them, laughing at them. Most uncool.

Divorce isn't as dismal as the hype would have us believe, either. Remember how we adapt to traditionally bad things too? Professor Lyubomirsky says that one study showed it takes around two years to adapt to (ie recover from) a divorce.

Forcing the random into a romcom shape

We try to overlay romcom endings on random life. We turn ordinary dumb luck, into extraordinary plot-writing.

'I'd finally made my peace with being single, and then *she* came along,' they beam, drunk on love intoxication.

Or, 'I'd just deleted all my dating apps, and then I bumped into him in the corner shop', as if he had been waiting in the wings for an entry cue.

No. Just no. This is guff, myth, fallacy, whereby once *we stop being so desperate*, and *we stop looking*, Cupid will throw us a bone (pun unintentional but what the hell, let's go with it).

We don't get sent people-shaped prizes by some cosmic reward system for finally being content single, we just so happen to meet someone through a friend or an app, who we hit it off with. It's just happenstance. A freakshake of circumstance, a backflip of serendipity.

Cupid is imaginary, he doesn't send out slings and arrows of romantic fortune. We are all just blundering through a fug of chance, sometimes crossing paths with people we fancy who fancy us back. That's all there is to it. I know that's ordinary as fuck, but it's also quite comforting in a peculiar way. Since it means there are many, many 'Ones'.

There is no fated love plot awaiting us. That idea is as fake as Universal Studios.

Dear childfree people

Choosing to be childfree is on the rise. I couldn't find any studies about men, bizarrely enough, but the Office of National Statistics recently released data showing that of women born in 1971, one in five of them is childfree at 45 (double that of those born in 1946). Yep. The childfree-ness has doubled.

The childfree (not child*less*) are often reported by studies to be happier overall, and yet they are relentlessly told they're missing out on one of the most transcendent life experiences of all.

I'm sure having a kid is wonderful, but I'm not into people telling me that my life lacks meaning, is a pale imitation of theirs unless I do, or I 'won't truly understand what love is' until I've procreated. I don't tell people who *have* children that they're 'missing out', or that they'll 'regret it'. There's a curious prejudice against the childfree.

In *Happy Ever After*, Professor Paul Dolan says that casting judgement on those who have strayed from the societal norm delivers a neuroscientific reward. 'There is now a range of brain imaging studies to show that we feel pleasure when we can punish those who do not conform to what we expect of them.'

Zoiks. Let's stop chasing the judgement buzz. Have a kid, have ten kids, adopt a kid, or don't have a kid; do whatever *you* want. Let's just all leave each other's life choices alone, 'kay?

It's high time that society begins to acknowledge that single people aren't crying into a microwave meal for one, while sad-swiping pictures of their married friends on Facebook.

Married is not best. Single is not best. Same with the kids/no kids debate. Neither is better, they're just *different*. And they have equal capacity to be joyful life choices.

SLACKER PARENTING

We are living throughout the refreshing ascent of the 'ordinary and proud' parent.

It's the reason the *Why Mummy Doesn't Give a Sh*t* book was a number one *Sunday Times* bestseller. Slummy Mummies have been replaced with Slacker Parents. Forget 'tiger mother'. This is the age of the 'sloth mum'. Superdad has been replaced with tongue-in-cheek blogs like 'Dad versus baby'.

When you have a baby, I have ascertained that bottomless reserves of patience, money and a desire to purée organic produce do not issue forth from your vagina along with the baby. Fathers' heads are not suddenly anointed with unlimited patience for decibel-smashing tantrums, or the ability to function pleasantly on four hours' sleep.

Parents are largely still the intolerant, skint, fond-of-fries-and-mayo people they were before; they just have a baby now.

I look on, agog, at the expectations of modern parents. Back in my childhood of Christmasses Past, I was lucky if my dad wasn't too pissed to remember to eat the cookies that I'd left for Santa, and to jingle some bells as I was drifting off. But now, my sister-in-law is utterly devoted to creating the most extraordinary Elf on the Shelf* scenarios.

When I was babysitting and needed to be in charge of the Elf, the only things I could think of was having the Elf graffiti 'Elf woz 'ere' on the bottom of the Connect 4, and to send him to a spa replete with a Rainbow Drop bath.

I'm not a parent, but I am an aunt to two, and unofficial aunt to many, and here's my observation, for what it's worth. Kids are mostly just fine as long as they're loved, warm and fed, even if they are wearing chocolate like warpaint or tirelessly defiant about not eating 'green fings'. They don't need a trampoline, they can just bounce around on the grass. A hose makes a better super-soaker than a £30 water pistol.

If you make them a delicious green curry (as my sister-in-law once did) you'll possibly receive the merciless criticism that it 'tastes like badgers, poo

---

* If you don't know about the Elf on the Shelf; the Elf toy is Santa Claus's spy, reporting back from each house on who is being naughty or nice. Dedicated parents have the Elf do something interesting every night in December, until Christmas Eve when Elf takes his naughty/nice report back to the North Pole. Elf is like Santa's behaviour tax auditor. I'm sure some kids would gladly stuff him into an incinerator given half a chance, but they're not allowed to touch him.

and limeade'. So don't bother. Embrace that which they will eat, like pizza with extra veggies, or Quorn spag bol, or tell them broccoli is actually tiny trees. 'Like a forest for dolls?' said five-year-old Maisy, suddenly lit up by the broccoli.

Persuade them that peas will give them the ability to slither like a snake, or bounce like a bunny; they know these are lies, but they collude in them anyhow. And if you're beating yourself up that they always choose ice cream over vegetables, know this: the only tastes kids are pre-programmed to prefer are sweet ones. It's not you and your failure as a sugar-restricting governor, it's just science.

I'm going to hand over to some actual parents now, since I'm shooting mostly in the dark here.

But I will finish by saying that I'm not sure what society asks of parents – to totally orbit another's needs above their own – is ever a good idea. As the cliché goes, put your own oxygen mask on first, gang. We all need me-time, kids included.

You don't have to fill their free time with crafting activities, or be a performing clown for their entertainment; it's said that 'unstructured playtime' is absolutely key to childhood development.

And nobody has an on-hand clown in adulthood, so you'll be teaching them the beauty of being bored, which I'm going to bang on about some more later.

Love to all the parents out there.

I don't know how you do it, and actually, maybe sometimes you don't have to.

'I went into parenting perfection overdrive'

By Grace Timothy, the author of *Lost in Motherhood: the memoir of a woman who gained a baby and lost her sh*t*

'When I found out I was unexpectedly pregnant I was fearful of the ordinary. I didn't tell anyone, but I was scared that after years of being fiercely ambitious at work, of trying to see all the best places and chasing the biggest dreams, motherhood would force me to relinquish all of those endless possibilities to a lifetime of cleaning, cooking and worst of all: school runs.

Then of course when my daughter arrived, my entire focus instantly shifted to her, and suddenly the mundane jobs I'd feared were lush; I loved her and I loved this new life.

But I was still set on perfection; it wasn't enough to be a good mum, I had to be perfect. I went into overdrive, doing what I imagined necessary for her to have the best life.

Protecting her from even the smallest discomfort, ensuring she was cognitively stimulated and read to, nourishing her with brain food, massaging her on the daily, teaching her to swim, schooling her at Baby Rhyme, socializing her with other kids *and* empowering her to be a feminist. All before she was a year old, obviously.

At the end of each day I would berate myself for not getting it right. I'd forgotten the changing bag, or not known how to lay her down for a sleep without her crying. I felt like I was letting her down by not having a clue. I stole a whole bunch of joy from myself by being so stressed.

The real joy kicked in once I embraced imperfection. I'd taken the foot off the pedal a little already out of sheer exhaustion. But then she had a health scare just after her second birthday, which proved that none of those spirited attempts at giving her the best life ever were going to stop bad things happening.

After the scare, we actually became way more relaxed. She was alive and well, which became my main source of joy. If we ended the day alive and loved, and hopefully clean and fed, we were doing OK.

In realizing the 'ordinary' was indeed good enough – and often preferable to my kid – I learned to forgive myself for my mistakes, to let go of my intense pursuit of perfection, and to instead strive for a loving, fun start to the life that she would mostly steer herself.

Right now my absolute favourite thing is watching TV with her. I get onto the sofa, make a nest of cushions around my body, and then she curls into the space under my arm. We eat crisps and cheese, and watch *Teen Witch* (which anyone who has seen will agree is not really suitable for an impressionable six-year-old).

There are no books being read during *Teen Witch*, no lessons being learned and probably very few memories being made. Sometimes there's very little talking too, beyond the odd faked fart and giggly yelp as I tickle her. I'm aware the school gate militia wouldn't approve.

But there's joy in that crumb-covered cuddle; both of us slack-jawed and entranced by a boy-obsessed witch with a bouncy perm. Magic.'

'Grand designs are a pointless exercise'

By Marcus Barnes, journalist
@mgoldenbarnes

'Even before our little blonde sweetheart, Marli, arrived I'd had the occasional thought that becoming a parent would present the perfect opportunity to create an exceptional human being. I mean, in my 38 years on this planet I've learned a hell of a lot.

"One day I'll be able to use all of my life experience to help my offspring become the best of the best," I'd think, unaware of the sheer arrogance contained in that statement.

How that knowledge and experience would be put to good use involved a wide range of methods, from New Age inspiration to more down-to-earth ideas, all of which would prepare our baby for its inevitable life as an extraordinary specimen.

Being a music lover, one of my main objectives was to play music to our unborn child in the womb. My mum told me that she had played music to me when I was a bump, my best friend and his wife played classical music to their unborn children and numerous online advice pieces recommended doing the same. We always have music on in the flat anyway, but I wanted more, I wanted to go beyond the ordinary ambient sounds of our music and do something spectacular.

One of our pals, who has an 18-month-old, told us he and his partner used a chime recommended by a sound healer friend of ours. Result! I got straight on to her and she pointed me in the direction of a beautiful, hand-crafted chime, which was set to the frequency of 'earth' (there are others available in the three remaining elements).

I wanted to play it to the bump every night, but that romantic ideal went out of the window as my partner and I worked late most nights, so were too tired to keep up the nightly mini sound bath. Hmm.

We'd also read that babies need to hear thousands of words every day to encourage their brain to develop. So I geared up to deliver a deluge of verbal diarrhoea as soon as she arrived. Once she was in my arms I would blabber, chat, sing and rap until I was out of breath, and then repeat that all day long. I even considered trying to record my daily word count somehow, crazy but it seemed to make sense during my plot to nurture a genius.

In the end, what Marli gets is the same as billions of babies all over the world: baby talk, silly noises, raspberries, cooing, repeated sounds ("bee" is one of my favourites) and infrequent conversations with her gurgling and me replying.

It's very early days but I'm learning fast that having grand designs as a parent is a pointless exercise. Despite your best intentions, any ambitious plans are dictated by time, energy and, of course, the baby. She doesn't need extraordinary treatment; life has been mindboggling enough for her from the get-go. The other day she was completely enchanted by the shadow of my hand dancing around the hood of her pram.

I'm settling into an enlightening truth: that the uncomplicated and ordinary is to be celebrated and embraced.'

'I want my kids to learn the joy of being ordinary'

By Kate Faithfull-Williams, well-being journalist and co-author of *The Feelgood Plan*
@katefaithfullwilliams

'Honestly, I never aspired to be an ordinary parent. Ordinary = average. I wanted to knock up courgette cakes from scratch, and to have my children beg for them. In public, while I faux blushed and other parents hid away their Mr Kipling packaging. I wanted to be Supermum.

Then I had kids, and discovered hypothetical parenting is so much easier than doing it IRL.

Picture me on a conference call in my office (the car) after the kids' swimming lessons. This is always a feral hour. My six-year-old has just got her first swimming badge and I've promised her a treat – a yellow rubber spider she's had her eye on.

I've lobbed a couple of bananas into the back seat, designed to silence chatter while I wind up this very important conference call about new calming magnesium supplements.

Fighting breaks out between my offspring. A traffic warden strolls towards the car. A bead of sweat grows on my top lip. I need a calming magnesium supplement more than anyone has ever needed anything ever.

I get the car into gear like a getaway driver towards the rubber spider shop before it closes, occasionally contributing an inane sentence to the magnesium conversation that will not die, because I'm Having It All.

I'm dragging the kids into the shop to claim the eldest's treat – their legs appear to have stopped working – and rushing my daughter through spider selection, still with one ear on the conference call. 'Why are you being like this, Mummy?' she wails, throwing herself down on the shop floor.

Good question: why? Everyone hates Supermum. Especially me.

So here's to giving up the charade. Here's to the precious breathing space that comes from not squeezing work into every minute of the day. Here's to the heavenly moment at the end of a playdate when you abandon wholesome craft projects and switch the TV on.

Let's celebrate fish fingers and sickening quantities of ketchup. Let's buy cupcakes with enough sugar to make us fly for the school bake sale, because the triumph of rocking up with a tin of homemade soggy courgette cakes and announcing, "I made these!" is overrated.

Yes, sometimes being ordinary feels like failing at parenthood. It feels slack, and "slack" is a word that no woman who has birthed a baby can hear without cringing. I have to forgive myself frequently: for snapping at the children, for changing the rules about bedtime, for looking at pictures of other people's kids on Instagram instead of being with my own, who are standing right in front of me demanding more snacks.

But, I don't want my daughters to put the same insane pressure on themselves as I put on me. I want them to learn the joy of being ordinary and doing ordinary things. Everyone is happier that way.'

So that covers *being* an ordinary parent, and forgiving yourself for it, but what about hanging onto all of those precious, fleeting, ordinary moments with them – rather than forgetting them, or underappreciating them, as we now know we are wont to do?

Kids are properly hysterical, on a daily basis. Tirelessly cute. You think you'll never forget what they just said or did, but you do. I find it extremely useful to now keep a rolling notes document on my phone of the priceless things my niece and nephew have said. Like how they deadpan, 'It's a shirt' or 'It's some Lego' before a friend has opened the present they've just given them.

I tap them in then and there, as otherwise they whoosh out of my head alarmingly quickly. Here are some recent entries of hilarities I have witnessed.

My nephew Liam: 'Mummy, have you heard of Bloody R Kip?'
His mum: 'I beg your pardon Liam.'
Liam: 'He wrote *The Jungle Book* and others.'
    His mum: 'Do you mean Rudyard Kipling?'

My niece Charlotte, playing doctors/patients with her friend.

Charlotte, as doctor: 'What's wrong with you then?'

Her friend: 'I've got a sore bum.'

'Doctor' Charlotte grimaces and thinks, hard.

'Sorry, I don't do bums.'

These moments are gold dust, and yet they blow away if we don't secure them, quicksmart.

NON-ITALIAN-WIDOW GRIEF

Grief often takes a different shape from that which we expect.

Before I actually lost someone incredibly close to me, I had a very specific expectation of grief. As a linear experience, drawing from unfathomable depths of sorrow, up into 'functioning, just about', and then ascending into some sort of renewed, if bittersweet, vigour for life.

When my bombastic father was taken aged just 65, care of the devastatingly fast reaper of lung cancer, it transpired that, just like everything else about me and my life, even my grief was ordinary. Pedestrian. No great shakes. It was very far from linear too. It came in fits and starts.

I had a night-day-night-day time lapse sequence in my head, of days spent in bed, takeaway cartons beside sympathy flowers, 87 unheard messages on the phone and living in a bathrobe.

But, it wasn't like that – at all. Given I still had bills to pay, deadlines to meet, a grumbling stomach to feed, shopping to do, a dog to walk, life just went on. I got dressed, shopped, exercised, made meals, talked to people, did my work, and fulfilled all but a few diary engagements.

Sleep would softly dismantle the news, so that in the morning, one, two, three…and my eyes would fill with tears as the realization reassembled its grisly self. But I got up, and got on with it, because that's just what we do. Within a week, I started knowing that my dad was dead even in the land between sleep and wakefulness. There was *no time* for the time lapse of extraordinary grief. Losing a parent was not, it turned out, the melodrama I expected, in which life screeched to a halt.

Plus, we had a godforsaken memorial to organize now, which involved getting half of his ashes from the Philippines to Ireland, and turned out to be a socially political nightmare where people were more awkward than supportive. Memorials, it turns out, are pretty much the same work and stress of a wedding, only everyone is really, really sad.

On the day of the memorial, I expected extravagant grief to cascade from me, unbidden, like a Mafioso's widow. But it didn't. I was so stressed out about the smooth running of the day, the unseen resentments circling like barracudas, the fact the sandwiches weren't out yet, the music being too quiet, that I totally overlooked my own chance to grieve.

From auto-grief to locked-in grief

I then entered what I can only describe as locked-in, exceedingly emotionally unintelligent grief.

At first, grief was a fait accompli. When I'd heard the news of his death, I had folded over and dropped my phone on the floor, as if right-hooked in the stomach by loss. I lay on the kitchen tiles, as expected, dominated by the overlord of bereavement.

Much as I'd expected, over the next few weeks, random things held the same indomitable sway. They had the power to pluck me from a workaday chore and plunge me into existential darkness, as if a soft animal grabbed by a claw and dropped into a chute.

The emerald of a pool table and thwack of the balls; Doc Martens (*Dad kicks them* 'Take those fecking things upstairs, howmanytimeshaveitoldyou'); the toasted-marshmallow dust of cinnamon lozenges; the sight of *any* bored father outside a changing room; the growl of a Subaru accelerating; Bruce Springsteen and stone wash jeans.

But then, the claw stopped airlifting me from my everyday and plonking me into the anguish chute. The auto-grief stopped, as I segued into the locked-in grief phase. The phase I'm still in now, whereby I constantly misdiagnose my grief.

I'll find myself sideswept by sorrow, and wonder why, and then remember it's Father's Day this weekend, so the 'Fathers!' advertising, social media and so on has worked its way into me undetected, like a mosquito bite, and is spreading. (I treated it by writing my dad a letter, comprised of all the things I'm aching to tell him. The sting subsided.)

An argument with a family member, money worries, disproportionate irritation when someone at work nicks your stapler. These can all be undiagnosed locked-in grief.

Grief doesn't just *happen*, I've found. You need to make it happen.

There are keys that unlock imprisoned grief; we just need to locate them. And use them, regularly. Otherwise that locked room becomes dank, cobwebbed, the keyhole rusts, and the things we need to air and unpack multiply, as if bewitched. Grief is something we need to schedule into our mental health must-do, just as we diarize counselling or Pilates.

Ordinary grief may be inconvenient in that it's incognito, a shapeshifter, and often shows up as something else. However, it means that life can occur around it. That you can lock yourself in a room and play loud Elvis Costello, or whatever song it is that makes your grief cascade. You can put on *The Big Lebowski* and allow yourself to come undone. Open a photo album and have it tumble out of you.

In a twisty-turny sort of way, I now find myself grateful for my ordinary, locked-in, undramatic grief. In the beginning, I thought it would be forever impossible for me to hear the song 'Romeo and Juliet' by Dire Straits without crying the kind of toddler cry whereby you struggle to breathe. But now I can. I thought I'd never be able to play Swingball, or smell a spliff, or eat snowballs, or see a rubber duck without losing my shit. But now I can. Which may not be a *joy*, but it sure is a relief.

Atheism and 'That's all, folks'

Being an atheist means that you have to make your peace with the prospect of a very ordinary death. For yourself, and your loved ones. One in four Brits now identifies as atheist, according to a 2018 British Social Attitudes survey; compared to just one in ten in 1998. Worldwide estimates say the number of atheists is approaching 500 million.

I've never felt convinced of the idea of a hereafter, not since I was a kid, when I believed in God mainly because I wanted to go to heaven rather than hell. My five-year-old brain's version of heaven resembled Care Bear land. Even though my parents didn't religiously attend church, I requested to go to Sunday School, because all my friends went, and I didn't want to miss out on Care Bear land.

Then, when the Care Bears started writing to me via the magical portal under my pillow, well, it was like God had started communicating directly with me, only in a hand that looked suspiciously like my mother's.

Now that I'm an adult, I almost wish I had faith, but I don't. Nonetheless, being an atheist doesn't mean I mope around life going 'well, we're going to die and that's it'. All I'll be doing after death, in my belief system, is pushing up daisies. It means that I know I only have one innings, that I best make the most of it, that this isn't a dress rehearsal, and that, to me, is invigorating. Atheism can be just as beautiful and profound a way to live – and die.

An unremarkable ash-scattering ceremony

We scattered Dad's ashes on Knockalla beach in Ireland, beneath Dad's favourite rally stage, which hairpins up the lush mountain. Our romantic expectations, you'll already have guessed, were very different to the reality.

As we walked onto the sunshine-streaked beach, a sped-up storm rolled in and whipped the waves and sand into a froth and swirl. We blundered into the wind. And when we eventually managed to dispense his ashes (there were *a lot* of ashes; also unexpected) into the North Atlantic, half of them blew back in our faces. Ash-scattering? More like ash-eating.

'Dad always had to have the last laugh!' we said to our wider family, waiting back in the car, as we marvelled at the storm outta nowhere. It would be lovely to think of my dad out there, riding on the back of a whale, summoning a storm with a wave of his cigarette; or his soul sitting in the belly of an oyster shell, his spirit churning in the wake of a fishing boat.

But, I don't believe he's out there, I believe he's gone. I have no 'here-ever-after' story to tell myself, no swaddle of the afterlife to curl up in.

Seagulls aren't ghosts, I don't think

Two years on from Dad's death, I have a particular seagull that keeps visiting my balcony – I've christened him Nigel. I talk to Nigel. I like Nigel. He's a dude. At first, he would look out to sea. But he soon started just staring directly into my flat, as if checking up on me.

Then the other day, I heard a strange thudding against the glass and found Nigel headbutting the patio door, trying to get in. I mean. I like Nigel a lot, but I'm not sure I'm ready for us to live together.

Two of my more spiritual friends are convinced this seagull is my late father. It's a nice idea. But in my belief system, Nigel is just a nosey, pushy 'gull. Not that I *know there isn't* an afterlife, of course I don't, I'm not omnipotent, no one knows for sure either way, but I do know that *I don't believe* there is.

Leonard Cohen put in his request for the afterlife just in case, 'I don't really understand that process called reincarnation but if there is such a thing I'd like to come back as my daughter's dog'. (I'd like to come back as one of those birds of paradise that do those hilarious mating dances.)

I don't believe my dad has come back as a seagull. But I still talk to the seagull sometimes as if it's him, because it feels good. It unlocks my grief, just as eating apple pie, or reading Donne's poetry does. And in bereavement, you take the good feels where you can find them.

Jamie Anderson, writer of a blog called *All My Loose Ends*, went viral with this quote: 'Grief, I've learned, is really love', wrote Jamie. 'It's all the love you want to give but cannot give. The more you loved someone, the more you grieve. All of that unspent love gathers up in the corners of your eyes and in that part of your chest that gets empty and hollow feeling. The happiness of love turns to sadness when unspent. Grief is just love with no place to go.'

I agree. It's energy that gets stuck and transmuted. With nobody to imprint upon, it turns inwards and glowers to anger, sadness and anguish. It's love that needs to go someplace; to light candles in churches, or incense at shrines, to cry to playlists, to bake birthday cakes for those no longer able to eat them. The love needs to run around, to dance, talk about the person, write letters to them and to hold honorary dinners. Grief needs a place to go.

'I would love to believe that when I die I will live again, that some thinking, feeling, remembering part of me will continue. But as much as I want to believe that, and despite the ancient and worldwide cultural traditions that assert an afterlife, I know of nothing to suggest that it is more than wishful thinking.'

Carl Sagan, *Billions & Billions: thoughts on life and death at the brink of the millennium*

ORDINARY JOYS PART III

- Fake flowers that look real, will last forever and weren't pulled by their ankles from their rightful home.

- When someone remembers your job interview, scary hospital appointment, or big pitch, and texts you to send good vibes.

- A chocolate biscuit dunked in English breakfast tea (served in a bone china cup, ideally). Un-ruddy-beatable.

- The invisible social contract that you are allowed to eat a family-sized portion of junk food in the cinema. Perhaps because it's dark.

- The snap-hiss-pull of opening a can and slaking your thirst.

- The 'wisdom and words' smell of bookshops.

- Skimming stones. Or, just hearing them *plunk* instead.

- Kids wearing noise-cancelling headphones at festivals. So cute I can hardly stand it.

- High-fiving and cheering marathon runners.

- Teasing a cat with a laser pen. The 'red dot' is their arch nemesis. Why can't they catch it and eat it? Why?! It's a feline mystery.

- The aural illusion of thinking you can hear the ocean in a sea shell.

- A fat, pale-faced harvest moon hanging out in the sky to watch the sunrise, like a person at a house party who refuses to go home.

....

....

....

....

....

V: ORDINARY EARNING

ODES TO THE ORDINARY

An ode to shite teenage jobs

The most common job done by today's teenagers is selling stuff online, said a survey of 3,000 students by Tutor House. They don't even leave the house in order to go to work. This makes me feel sad, because I, like all people of a certain generation, think that *the way we did it was the best way*.

My first Saturday job was, strictly speaking, illegal. I was 13, so younger than the official 'can start working' age of 14 of that time. I worked in a hairdresser for £1-an-hour, washing hair and trying valiantly not to get water down little old ladies' faces (and failing, thus being taken off hair-washing duty when one too many sexagenarians left with her eye make-up down to her chin).

So, I was demoted to sweeping the wisps of unwanted hair, but most of my duties took place in a windowless basement room; washing and drying towels, and arranging dyes into order.

But, I liked it. I liked the sharp smell of hair dye, the banter of the bleached'n'manicured staff, the feeling of responsibility. When they gave me a tenner cash at the end of my shift, I felt the adult thrill of reaping the monetary rewards of my towel-based toils.

Denzel Washington and Beyoncé were right there with me, on the hair sweeping as one of their first jobs. Madonna worked at a Dunkin' Donuts. Taylor Swift had to pluck praying mantis pods off Christmas trees, so they didn't hatch in people's houses. George Clooney sold insurance door-to-door before he hit the big time. Calvin Harris date-rotated sandwiches in Marks & Spencer.

The washing of towels gig meant that when I landed a Saturday job at the very ordinary Boots in Chelmsley Wood shopping centre, I felt like Queen of the World (the only thing Chelmsley Wood was ~~famous~~ infamous for, was starring in a show about the growing prevalence of girl gangs. I once let the kingpin of a gang nick loads of make-up, rather than have her kick my head in). Boots were less chuffed about my appointment, given I wagged about one Saturday in four due to waking up in random places wearing squashed sequins, clutching a can of cider and with cigarette ash in my hair.

Everything is relative, in the world of work, and spending a year or so in a windowless basement gains you a greater appreciation of being able to see sunlight later on.

JETTISONING 'PRESENTEEISM'

> 'Whether you're Gordon Brown or the bloke pushing a
> broom down the street, we are all nagged by an inner voice
> which says that we're underachieving, that if we just put our
> shoulder to it more, we could make the breakthrough that
> resolved our lives...it's a delusion, a crustacean-like psychic
> defence against reality. "You could rule the world", our
> psyches tell us, "if only you worked harder."'
>
> John Naish, *Enough: breaking free from the world of excess*

The cult of 'presenteeism' is currently stapling us to our desks, as if with a giant stapler. 'Stay there! If you leave, we will think you are a bad employee!' Doing your ordinary set hours is seen as audacious, outdated and most certainly slack. 'She leaves at 5.30 on the dot, every day,' goes the watercooler tongue-wag. The temerity!

Last year, an alarming Total Jobs survey discovered that almost a third of British bosses expect their employees to do more hours than they're contracted to do, with IT and tech workers the most likely to be expected to work late. The UK capital of presenteeism is – Birmingham.*

Almost half of all workers in Birmingham stay late for fear of being judged for buggering off at 5.30pm. Even if they have no work to do. And when people earn big (over £50K), six in ten of them feel fraught with worry about the idea of leaving when the clock ticks to hometime.

More hours lead to *less* productivity

This nonsense is a peculiarly British (and American) attitude. But your boss is *wrong*. Longer hours don't necessarily lead to more productivity. In fact, it often has the opposite effect.

A 2017 article in *Time* published a fascinating table from OECD*, which

---

* I know you just said that in your head in a Brummie accent. 'Burrrrr-ming-umm'. Which isn't annoying for people from Birmingham *at all*.

showed that the world's most productive countries put the least hours in. Of the 35 countries analysed, *all of* the countries whose workers averaged less than 30 hours a week made it into the top ten. Notably Luxembourg (which was top), Norway, Denmark, Belgium, the Netherlands, Germany and France.

In fact, seven of the top ten 'most productive' countries, put the *least* work hours in. As you trace your finger down the chart, there's a notable trend of productivity swan diving as the hours increase. Huh.

Meanwhile, in terms of taking holiday, US workers are infamous for often not taking their allotted days for annual leave; which is something Brits are now beginning to mimic, lemming-like. 'Let's all walk repeatedly into this brick wall.' *Bash, bash, bash*

A third of Brits don't take their holiday entitlement, to the tune of four days a year. Four days when we could have been sandy-toed on a beach, but we chose to force our feet into work shoes instead. Madness.

Elsewhere, they've wised up and stopped walking en masse into the wall of brain-bashed burn out. The *Financial Times* reported that an enormous German company, Daimler, has now given circa 100,000 employees the option to nominate an alternative contact in their out-of-office, and then auto-delete any emails that come in. Meaning they come home from annual leave to an empty inbox. In the UK, we tend to put our out-of-office on, but reply anyway.

In France, it became employment law in 2017 that companies have to give their workers a 'right to disconnect'; as in, they're not expected to answer work emails outside of office hours. *And* their lunches can legitimately last up to two hours. *C'est magnifique.*

When I lived in Belgium, I noticed that I was almost never asked 'What do you do?', whereas in England, it is always among people's top questions. Where do you live, what do you do, are how Brits get to know each other (or, you could argue, know where to pin each other on the working/middle/upper classboard). In Belgium, people work to live, rather than the other way around, so your job is one of the least interesting things about you.

Our in-built concentration checkpoint

We're not meant to do extraordinary amounts of work. Which is why we have an inbuilt liminal point of concentration, a natural threshold when our brain

---

* Organisation for Economic Co-operation and Development. (The next footnote will be more fun, I promise.)

just stops working. 'Surely, if it was advantageous for us to be able to laser focus for ten-hour stretches, that would have evolved, right?' asks Professor Cregan-Reid, who specializes in evolution.

'However, still, even after two million years of our species evolving, our concentration falters at around four to five hours. We get to a point where we just can't do it anymore,' he says. 'There's a very good reason evolution has kept that concentration checkpoint.'

For a start, we need to stay socially engaged with other people, so it's our body forcing us to go do that. 'But also, if Johnny of the savannah was transfixed by a beetle pushing a mound of dung for hours on end, he was more likely to have a predator creep up on him,' points out Cregan-Reid. Obviously, we're not likely to be stalked by wild creatures if we're in a monomanic work flow, but our body still wants us to eat, rest, chat.

'Current guidance is that we should stop every 50 minutes for a five to ten minute break and execute a completely different task,' he adds. 'Yet our bosses would choke on their muesli if they saw us doing this.'

In Britain and the USA, we labour under a 'more hours, more productivity' myth. Much like a packhorse toiling under an extra-heavy plough, when there's a much lighter one languishing by the side of the field, that would do a better job.

'Less hours, more productivity' is the data-proven reality. An ordinary amount of work, a lower amount of hours, is actually the unexpected ideal, both for us, and our bosses.

ODES TO THE ORDINARY
An ode to not driving

I have a unique perspective when it comes to driving, given I did not even attempt to drive a car until I was 37.

When I turned 18, my mum and stepdad gave me £500 and said, 'We strongly suggest you spend this on driving lessons.' So I spent it on tiny outfits, clubbing, pints of cider and packets of cigarettes. Instead of going driving, I went raving, to nights that sounded like they were named after astronauts' food – Spacehopper, Atomic Jam, Cosmic Bass.

I have still not passed my driving test. I tried last year, and failed. Why did I fail? Oh, nothing too serious. Just a cataclysmic and potentially fatal lapse in judgement.

At the end of my test, the examiner broke it to me, 'So, overall, that was a good drive. You only got three minor faults out of 15. But I'm afraid I'm going to have to fail you. Given I can't ignore the fact that at one point you were on the wrong side of the road.'

Wrong side of the road?! What? 'I think you thought you were still in the one-way system we'd just been through,' he said, kindly.

So, I have never driven a car, other than during lessons. And it's a bit of a trend. Experts think we hit 'peak car' in the 1990s; 34 per cent of twentysomethings now don't have a driving licence. Over four in ten new learners are now over 25.

In places like Australia, NZ, Canada and the US, the mind-boggling vastness of the land, and the inconvenience of cross-country public transport, has kept youngsters driving, but in Britain, many are now opting not to bother.

Personally, my very delayed learning is down to three key things. Living in London for most of my adult life, where you pretty much only get a car once you have kids.

Secondly, my fear of wielding a deadly weapon.

And thirdly, being an easily distracted fantasist, which resulted in my once flying off a bike and faceplanting in San Francisco, due to having seen a particularly fetching painted lady of a house. Martin Amis once wrote, 'Poets don't, can't, shouldn't drive' and while I'm not saying I'm a poet, I definitely have the daydream-prone leanings of one.

I have long felt like a giant lumbering kidult for not being able to drive, but now, my pathological determination to find the good in all 'bad' means that I have alighted upon the many perks of not driving.

I can choose to either bemoan the fact that when I travel my space and ears are invaded by other people, rather than being enclosed in a bubble whereby I choose the sounds and smells. Or I can pluck out the plusses.

1. I believe that while driving, you're not allowed to read, it's frowned upon to people watch and that staring out of the window is definitely not permitted. All things which are immensely enjoyable about public transport, or being a passenger.

2. It also means I walk for at least an hour a day, which apparently means I'm 21 per cent more likely to live until I'm 90, according to one 2019 Netherlands study.

3. Finally, driving brings with it the untold stress and expense of parking. When I show up somewhere, I just walk in. I don't have to drive around endlessly to find a place to dispense my hunk o' metal while dozens of others do the same; nor do I have to engage in 'that's my space, dickwad' parking-rage politics or faff about with pay-and-display machines that defy all logic.

I'm sure driving pleasure shall, at some point, be mine. I've already experienced the satisfaction of crushing a parallel park, and the stomach-elevator thrill of cresting a hill (something you curiously don't experience as a passenger), but for now, I'm more than happy to carry on reading and staring out of windows.

If you're with me on the non-driving, whether it be from a lack of licence, or a licence but no automobile, you can look at your car-free existence in one of two ways.

Either as an abject failure to launch. Or that you are a stealth eco-warrior whose carbon footprint is probably the size of a toddler's Converse. I choose the latter, these days.

WHY BIG EARNING DOESN'T MEAN BIG HAPPINESS

'It is not the man who has too little, but the man who craves more, that is poor.'

Seneca

When you type 'I want to be' into Google, it suggests the following: 'A ninja' (don't we all, Daniel-san), 'Alone' (presumably powered by Greta Garbo admirers), 'With you' (awwww), 'A billionaire' (Uh-huh) and finally in fifth place, 'Happy'.

For the purposes of this chapter, let's ignore the others, and take on the 'I want to be a billionaire' desire.

'If only I could earn six figures, I'd be so much happier,' is the oft-heard lament over sundowners in British pubs. We long to roll around on a goose-down bed full of cash, thinking fistfuls of fifties will provide the answers to all of our woes.

If a kingfisher-blue genie appeared in front of me right now, wisping out of my water bottle, I would wish for a million pounds, in a heartbeat. Extraordinary riches, please genie.

But, that isn't necessarily wise, on my part. Or anyone's part. If I had a pound for every study I've now seen that pierces the myth that high rollers have higher happiness I would, ironically, be quite rich.

Rising wages mean less well-being

The leading expert in the salary/happiness correlation (arguably, but it's my book, so...) is psychologist, Professor Ed Diener, who cites studies which reveal 'that rising wages predict less well-being', showing a spike in divorce rates, stress and a puncturing of the enjoyment of small activities. Yikes.

When we look at a graph of happiness levels related to income, we see a perfect arc. Happiness levels are low at the low points – and at the higher levels. 'Happiness goes up with increases in income at the lower end of the distribution, but then it falls with higher incomes,' confirms Professor of Behavioural Science, Paul Dolan in his book, *Happy Ever After*.

The peak happiness, the crest of the arc, is seen between $50K and $75K, or in British terms at the time of going to press, between around £40K to £59K.

'People who earn between $50K and $75K experience more pleasure and more purpose than any other income group,' says Professor Dolan.

The latest figures from the Office of National Statistics found that the average Brit who works full-time earns just over £35K, so not far off the 'peak happiness' crest of the arc.

In other results gathered by a gigantic Gallup study undertaken in 2008 by a Nobel-prize-winning psychologist (among others), they asked 450,000 Americans, and found that 'beyond about $75,000/y, there is no improvement whatsoever in any of the three measures of emotional well-being'.

A low salary is obviously not good either, with this study concluding that 'lack of money brings both emotional misery and low life evaluation... however, higher income is neither the road to experienced happiness nor the road to the relief of unhappiness or stress'.

'Contrary to what most of us might expect, those earning over $100K are no happier than those with incomes of $25K. And it's worse for rich folk when we look at purpose,' continues Professor Dolan in *Happy Ever After*. 'Those with the highest incomes report the least purpose in their experiences.'

What does this mean? CEOs are no happier than their PAs. In fact, they might be *less* happy.

The Trojan horse of money

'Mo money, mo problems' is bang on the money. Money is the ultimate Trojan horse of a gift. Holy shit, what a cool gift! And then all of these marauders crawl out of it in the dead of night.

Why? I think because as the digits on your pay cheque rachet upwards, so do the ballache of tax returns, nutty things like 'breakfast meetings' (read: working before work begins), the stress of manhandling huge budgets, plummeting investments, managing stroppy staff (actual hell, in my experience), placating tenants, having to be available even while on holiday, people trying to get that money off you (even family and friends). Money comes with a long list of side effects that really aren't fun, but are largely inevitable if you want to tread the corridors of power wallpapered with fifties.

'Economists have found that two-thirds of the benefits of a raise in income are erased after just one year, in part because our spending and new "needs" rise alongside it,' says Professor Lyubomirsky. We begin to hang out with people who earn a similar amount. 'We get used to – and perhaps even "addicted" to – the higher standard of living,' she adds.

We tend to adjust our tastes to our income, so suddenly you want gourmet fish and chips, or nitro cold brew coffee, or for everything you wear to be Whistles or Reiss, so you spend a heap more money and only have slightly better fish suppers, coffee and clothes.

Money is like a haughty cat

Obsessing about your bank balance screws with your happiness. Seriously.

'People should understand that placing great emphasis on the acquisition of wealth can be counterproductive to happiness, and that gaining increased income has dangers as well as pleasures,' a report Professor Ed Diener co-authored cautions.

What is true, however, is that those who are happy to begin with, tend to wind up with fatter treasure-chests. A study called 'Beyond Money: Toward an Economy of Well-Being' said, 'People who report that they are happy subsequently earn higher incomes than people who report that they are not happy, a finding that calls into question the direction of causality between income and well-being'.

We've got it all back to front. We think that money makes us happy, but it's the other way round: we attract money *when* we're happy.

Put those two things together. It seems that fixating on money nixes our happiness – and in tandem, the chances of us actually getting more of it. What a mischievous joke the universe has played on us.

It's like how if you want to attract a haughty cat, pet wisdom says you have to ignore said cat, and just concentrate on hanging out with your friends, since then it will assume you're the Alpha. And come and infinity-sign around your legs in a bid to win your Alpha blessing.

If we concentrate on being happy, rather than being rich, riches are actually more likely to come forth.

Are lottery-winners happier than your average bear?

In 1978, a trio of American researchers famously spearheaded a study whereby they measured the happiness levels of lottery winners contrasted with a control group (who didn't win a sausage). They were surprised to discover that lottery winners were only infinitesimally happier than the control group a year after their win. Lottery-winners' happiness rolled in at 4 out of 5 as opposed to the 'non-winners' average of 3.82, a difference so negligible that the study's authors asserted 'lottery winners were not happier than controls'.

As the authors of the study summed it up, 'Eventually, the thrill of winning the lottery will itself wear off…gradually even the most positive events will cease to have impact'.

This same study also spliced the relative happiness of golden-ticket-holders against those who had endured catastrophic accidents and were now paraplegic. What they found was compelling. When the two groups were asked to rate the pleasure they derived from everyday activities (what they called 'mundane pleasures') such as chatting with a friend, watching telly, laughing at a joke, or receiving a compliment, the accident survivors felt more happiness from these incidental, daily joys, than the lottery-winners did.

The control group of non-winners also felt significantly more pleasure in the 'mundane pleasures', than the ones who now had conspicuous wealth. It seems that just as our tastes match our income, our expectations do too, meaning that the mega-rich derive very little pleasure from the perfectly lovely humdrum.

Kanye is just as pissed off as you are

Take Kanye West, for instance. 'Rich people don't necessarily have less negative emotions just because they live in privilege', says neuroscientist Dr Korb.

Kanye has just as many problems as you emotionally; you're upset because your bus is late, but he's equally as upset that his chauffeur is a minute late. It just takes a lot less to vex him, because he expects a lot more. Envisage a fixed range of emotion, set from 'vexed – pleased', going up a chart of expectations. Kanye et al's 'vexed – pleased' slider is located higher up. It takes more to please, and less to vex.

If you eat at Nobu the whole time, a standard sushi restaurant is going to leave you cold. If you're used to silky Egyptian cotton, ordinary-yet-wholesome cotton will feel scratchy. Kanye et al think they have it made, but all their extraordinary existence is doing, is slaying the joy of ordinary things.

I was once randomly upgraded to first class on a flight to America. The opulence was staggering; there was an art deco bar, roomy showers, crystal and linen, and I even had a shoulder massage mid-flight. I wore that exact same outfit to the next five flight check-ins, but no cigar; I never got randomly upgraded again. And guess what that deluxe one-off did to the five following flights? Made them *less pleasurable*. I was less chuffed about the just-out films and guilt-free reading time than I usually would have been.

I'm not imagining the comedown. A 2014 study by Harvard psychologists called 'The Unforeseen Costs of Extraordinary Experiences' turned up the finding that, 'participants thoroughly enjoyed having experiences that were superior to those had by their peers, but having had such experiences spoiled their subsequent social interactions and ultimately left them feeling worse than they would have felt if they had had an ordinary experience instead'. In a nutshell, what goes up must come down. We may be exuberant in the narcotic first-class moment, but there's an extraordinary hangover awaiting us.

Finally, if you need any more convincing that money can't buy happiness, no sirree, then this should seal the deal. 2018 data found that the planet's three happiest countries are far from the richest (Finland, 37th on the wealth scale, and Denmark and Norway, respectively 25th and 26th). Here in the UK, we are fourth on the wealth index, yet sit 15th on the happiness scale.

The US may be top dog in wealth stakes, but their happiness languishes at 19th. Outdoorsy New Zealand isn't exactly flush at 21st on the rich list, yet their well-being is aglow at 8th place.

Meanwhile Canada and Australia are less extreme, and pretty balanced with respect to their wealth/mental health ratings. Canada rolls in at 7th for money and 9th on happiness; while Aussies feature 8th for wealth, and 11th for contentment.

Sinfully rich people who live just like us

Many of the planet's millionaires know that money can't buy them happiness, they know that contentment is more about giving than getting, so they are either intent on giving most of their riches away, or determined to live just as they did before they landed on the Rich List.

Keanu Reeves supposedly gave away £50 million of his earnings from *The Matrix* franchise to the unsung heroes of the cast; the costume and special effects teams. He's frequently papped on the subway and browsing sales racks. And has been quoted as saying, 'Money is the last thing I think about. I could live on what I have already made for the next few centuries'.

Shailene Woodley exclusively buys second-hand clothes and makes her own deodorant out of baking soda, coconut oil, pepper and lavender essential oil. Sarah Jessica Parker has been quoted saying she makes her son wear hand-me-downs.

Mark Zuckerberg drives what he calls a 'not ostentatious' Acura, which costs $30K; an expensive car for most of us, but is the equivalent of a Lada for a billionaire. He has also signed The Giving Pledge, which means he gives over half of his earnings to charity.

The legendary architect Antoni Gaudí, he of Barcelona's astonishing Sagrada Família, lived so simply, and dressed so humbly, that he was mistaken for a peasant at the end of his life.

Jeff Buckley knew that money couldn't buy happiness too. In 'Satisfied Mind', Buckley sings that money can't buy back your youth when you're old, a friend when you feel lonely, or peace within your soul. 'The wealthiest person, is a pauper at times, compared to the man with a satisfied mind,' the song goes.

As Fearne Cotton neatly writes in *Happy*, 'I watched the sunset in many countries, climbed mountains, partied until the birds sang and did jobs that seemed so much bigger than me. I feel so lucky to have experienced these moments in my life, and fun and joy were definitely woven throughout them, but they weren't teleporting me to the island of happiness like I had hoped.'.

Higher earners moan more

A study wryly entitled 'Stressed out on four continents' discovered that moaning about busyness comes disproportionately from those earning higher incomes, 'partly because their members choose to work more hours, partly too because they have higher incomes to spend during the same amount of non-work time'. Oh no, I have no time to spend all my money! Is the upshot.

'Getting rich doesn't mean you will receive a special bonus and your days will become 25 hours long instead of 24,' says the very sage Fumio Sasaki, in his book *Goodbye, Things: the new Japanese minimalism*.

Actually, what getting rich means, is that you have aeons more to do and less time to actually do it. There's a notion that you will be able to loll around being fed grapes, and waving for one of your minions to play the harp, but the reality is not like that.

Extraordinary riches come with extraordinary stress. I don't know about you, but finding all of this out has made me very happy with where I am, thanksallthesame.

'Our entire life we chase the wrong things because we think having more money and buying more stuff will make us more happy. But it doesn't. You know why a billionaire has 100 Ferraris? Because 99 weren't enough.'

Oliver Markus Malloy

ODES TO THE ORDINARY
An ode to Millennials

I think 'Millennialism' is the new prejudice. We give them such a rough time.

Before you dismiss me as a snowflake-sympathizer who will probably melt into my own tears while on a liberal march, take a look at some of these headlines from mainstream press:

MILLENNIALS HAVE OFFICIALLY RUINED BRUNCH

MILLENNIALS WANT MONEY, BUT NOT HARD WORK

HOW MILLENNIAL LACK OF MANNERS IS KILLING CLASS

And my personal favourite:
MILLENNIALS ARE KILLING THE NAPKIN INDUSTRY

Bret Easton Ellis, the objectionable writer of *American Psycho*, dubbed those born between 1982 and 1996 'Generation Wuss' and was pictured beside the headline, 'What is Millennial culture? There's no writing. None of them read books'.

Here's the truth about Millennials. They bring enormously needed tech-y skills to the workplace. They care so much that they go on protests. They are appalled by the 'isms' we have put up with/perpetuated for so long. They have more education under their belts than any generation in our history. They went through adolescence being tagged on socials having been filmed/videoed at their worst (and didn't have nervous breakdowns). They know what 'meta' means and use it with verve and an arched eyebrow. I have no clue when something is 'meta', even though I know the definition of it.

Also, although I have read alarming surveys which show that Millennial men still think men are smarter academically (despite women in their class getting better grades), and that women should still shoulder most of the housework, a more encouraging 2017 study found that Millennial men are just as likely (one in two) as Millennial women to describe themselves as 'feminists'. Brilliant.

They know that 'feminist' is just another word for 'equalist'. Like Germaine Greer once said, 'We are not feminists because we hate men. We are feminists because we respect and love men, and we do not understand why they do not always return that respect'.

I walked down the street earlier today behind a stone-cold fox wearing tight white jeans. We walked past six men. I watched with interest, like an anthropological observer.

The three Millennials glanced at her – their eyes widened in shock at her extraordinary beauty – and then they looked away. The three non-Millennials (aged between 40 and 80) openly stared at her chest and crotch, and then swivelled to unabashedly get a rear-view shot, as if she were free, walking porn.

I'm not saying this is representative of all Millennials and non-Millennials, I mean, it was a sample size of six men forgodsake, but it just backs up what I've observed in my lived experience. Even I was objectifying white-jean vixen more than the Millennial men.

Had she walked down Birmingham's Broad Street in the early noughties, she would have been grabbed and thrown over some geezer's shoulder. I think things are getting better, perhaps because transgressions are now more vocalized.

If Millennials are 'snowflakes', I think this is apt since snow is pretty good at covering up ugliness. Our only hope to save the planet may well be our substantially non-drinking, vegan-eating, bike-riding Millennials. They are likely the solution to the eco-geddon we are torpedoing towards on a cloud of carbon. Many Millennials are so 'woke' that they often make the rest of us look practically catatonic.

Millennials, I love you.

BUSY AS A BADGE OF HONOUR

Extraordinarily busy: good.

Ordinary busy: bad. Idling at life. Needs to put pedal to metal more!

Right? This is our cultural belief, that tentacle-arms its way into our work lives and social lives, scribbling way too many things into our calendars whenever we're not looking. You need to legitimately be doing something, in order to be permitted to say no to something else. It's bananas.

And then we get too busy, and belly-ache about being busy. I just accidentally right-clicked on 'busy' in this manuscript and Word suggested 'FREQUENT. Consider revising'. Thanks Word, for pointing out that I bang on about being busy so dang much.

It's a scourge, this bleating about how busy we are, hence headlines like 'Being busy "new badge of honour"' (*The Times*) and 'This busy-bragging epidemic must be stopped. If only we could find the time' (touché, the *Guardian*).

I think one of the reasons it's endemic in the modern condition to bleat on about how busy we are, is because of the mostly invisible nature of our busyness.

Our foremothers and forefathers used to be bombing around like harried bluebottles, doing actual physical things like feeding sheep and going to markets and hand-delivering letters and Chaucer-knows-what-else. You could *see* how busy they were.

While on my busiest days, this is what you'll see if you look at me:

Me, inert, staring unblinkingly at a computer, my spine a touch too straight, as if someone has indeed rammed a pole up my ass.

I don't even have a mouse with an audible click now to 'clickety-click' denote my urgent stuff-doing. I'll occasionally bash at my keyboard for a while, just to make the point that I'm *so busy*, but most of it is just me staring at a screen. For all the watcher knows, I'm looking at a *Buzzfeed* round-up of animals doing hilarious things.

Being busy sitting is the new smoking

Indeed, sitting for such long periods of time has been declared the new smoking by experts in *The Lancet*.

We all sit down for an average of 10 to 15 hours a day and bun fight for a seat on the train/in a bar even after we've been sat down all day. We're obsessed with sitting down. When the irony is, the person doing the best by their body, is the one who doesn't get a seat.

'We're in an evolutionary blip as a result,' says Professor Cregan-Reid. 'Life expectancy is now static rather than rising. In 100 or 200 years I think future generations will look back and go, "I can't believe how lazy they were!" One of the ironies of sedentary life is that people's fingers roam one to two miles a day across their keyboards. If only we did that with our feet.'

Cregan-Reid points out that bad backs are a relatively new ailment, borne of all this sitting down. No mention of them appears in Shakespearean times; it wasn't until the early 19th century that they start appearing in literature. 'More than half of those who experience lower back pain spend their working day seated,' he says.

My grandparents owned a sweet shop and a petrol station, so they stood up constantly. My grandpa was walking miles a day even into his eighties, so my spinal future is likely to look different to his, even though I exercise frequently, for one simple reason: I sit down a hellofa lot more than he did.

We may be sitting down way more, but we're just as busy, even though we look less busy. For those of us with computer-based jobs (please excuse us for a moment or two, butchers, bakers and candlestick-makers) we are carrying out much the same work as our ancestors, but just with a lot less tangible *doing*.

We are sending emails, where once they had physical face-to-face meets; doing grocery shopping online, where once they trawled farmer's markets*; paying bills, where once they went to the post office to do so. It means we leave work just as intellectually tired, but physically wired, since during all of our busyness we actually barely moved.

So, basically, the only way to let people know how busy we are now, is to tell them all the bloomin' time, until they're sick to the back teeth of us doing so. Le sigh.

---

* They quaintly called them 'markets'.

Multi-tasking is worse than smoking a spliff

When we're busy, we try to slay a dozen tasks with the same hour.

And yet, trying to multi-task dings our IQ. A UCL study which looked at 80 clinical trials found that the IQ of those who try to juggle messages and work fell by 10 points. This is the equivalent to not sleeping the night before. AT ALL. And over double the IQ drop you would experience if you smoked a spliff.

They neatly named the study, 'Text and email reduces IQ more than cannabis'. When we're busy, we tend to check our email more, when actually, we need to check it *less*. Next time you pull your phone out in the middle of a humdinger of a task, for a 'break', remember that you'd actually be better off sparking up a reefer, in terms of the intellectual price tag.

But largely, our busy level is our choice. Aside from working/single parents, who are our modern day superheroes, most of us have an option as to our busy levels. I will often bemoan how busy I am and then remember, hang on, I said yes to dog-sitting, plus my full-time job, plus all of these social engagements. Me. Nobody strong-armed me into it.

I keep inviting people to stay for the weekend, so why am I surprised when they do. I choose to clean the entire flat before they do so, they don't *make me*. I want to make nice meals, which takes work. My busy level is my choice.

Given I suffer from the delusion that I can bend time, I frequently take on too much work. Usually, my body tells me first. I went through a period recently when I got three colds in six months, when I was ill twice in five *years* before that.

I cleared my social diary to purely focus on work. Five 10–14 hour work days later, I still didn't feel on top of things. I found myself sobbing in the toilet after yoga because my yoga teacher had asked, 'Are you...OK?' (Yogis, man. They have emotional x-ray.)

Cue these recurring thoughts. 'If I just work a bit more, I'll do better!' The voice whispered, 'Maybe you're lazy, rather than busy'. However, I don't roll like that anymore. I try to self-parent, even though it's still not a natural instinct. I looked at ways to lighten my load, rather than berate myself for buckling beneath it.

We all need help sometimes. Whether it's a favour from a family member, or one of those recipe-delivery services, or a tumble dryer, or an 'I'll get back to you but here are some FAQs' autoreply, or telling a friend you're in a bad place. Stoicism is over-rated.

What are we busy about?

Now that I have gotten my busy levels down to a medium level, an ordinary nicety, here are my golden rules of keeping it this way:

1. 'Do I really need to do this right now?' Given that I am prone to do bonkers stuff like sort the drawers that time forgot when I have loads of more urgent things to be getting on with.

2. I under- rather than over-promise (over-promising is a knee-jerk tic of my people-pleasing).

3. I say 'no' and then have to jump up and down to rid myself of how wretched it makes me feel.

As Henry David Thoreau said, '…it is not enough to be busy. So are the ants. The question is what we are busy about.' Allowing the busy-whirl to subside and spin to a blurry-coloured stop is important.

ODES TO THE ORDINARY
An ode to common-or-garden procrastinating

One in five of us, research says, is not just a procrastinator; we are 'chronic procrastinators'. Eep.

I recently had a motherload of a time-sensitive task to get stuck into. So instead, I watched four hours of *Killing Eve*. Did it feel good? A little, when I was dropping popcorn into my mouth piece-by-piece having stowed my laptop safely out of sight under the sofa.

But overall?

No, because I had that gnaw that accompanies all procrastination. That 'I shouldn't be doing this, I should be doing that' thrum of guilt.

When I finally stop reaching for distraction, and start the huge undertaking hanging over me like a shipping container swaying on ropes, it always feels so good. We're told procrastinating is fun, but in my experience it's *really not*. It's like sleeping with someone you know doesn't respect you. It's shame-fun. It's pleasurable, and yet horrible at the exact same time.

So, now I outwit my ordinary urge to procrastinate, with these hacks:

1. Simply denying the whisper
Answering the call of procrastination is a self-perpetuating prophecy in the habit centre of the brain (the dorsal striatum), says Dr Korb. 'Whenever the voice whispers something, and you do it, you make it stronger and harder to ignore,' he says. 'This is just how the dorsal striatum works.'

Some part of the obligation we're avoiding has created an unpleasant feeling, he says. 'So we seek out distraction to avoid the unpleasant feeling,' whether it's a film, or a run or a phonecall. 'The distraction releases dopamine, but as soon as it ends, those unpleasant feelings rise up again,' says Dr Korb. 'So what do you do now? Reach for more distraction. Because it worked before.'

The more you deny procrastination, the better you get at denying it.

2. The five-minute oven timer
Kevin Systrom may be CEO and co-founder of Instagram – but he's still susceptible to procrastination. And so he has come up with a simple trick.

'If you don't want to do something, make a deal with yourself to do at least five minutes of it. After five minutes, you'll end up doing the whole thing,' he recently told Axios.

Using the oven timer is perfect for this hack. Once it *dings*, you generally have the bit between your teeth and are ready to gallop on.

3. Taking it a bird at a time

As per the advice of the inimitable Ann Lamott. 'Thirty years ago my older brother, who was ten years old at the time, was trying to get a report on birds written that he'd had three months to write,' writes Lamott, in her book *Bird by Bird: some instructions on writing and life*.

'[It] was due the next day. We were out at our family cabin in Bolinas, and he was at the kitchen table close to tears, surrounded by binder paper and pencils and unopened books on birds, immobilized by the hugeness of the task ahead. Then my father sat down beside him, put his arm around my brother's shoulder, and said, "Bird by bird, buddy. Just take it bird by bird".'

This saves me, constantly. I just take it a bird at a time.

4. Making it so small, I can't say no

I think I pinched this from Gretchen Rubin, but when I have a monstrous task overfacing me, plunging me into daunting shadow, I now break it down into absurdly tiny pieces. 'Print X out.' 'Call Y person.' 'Send an email to Z.'

Once the tasks are miniscule, I can no longer say no to them. I can press 'print' on a document, for pity's sake. It works.

5. The minute-bubble trick

Another thing I find useful, is putting circles next to tasks, in which I write down how long they will take. Often, the tasks I push back the most, are actually things that take less than ten minutes. For instance, I have been putting off measuring and ordering blinds for my bedroom for, oh, almost a *year*. Thanks to my fondness for gauzy, fairy-wing pretty curtains, my room is 'brighter than heaven' (one guest said) come sunrise. What finally made me do this extremely simple task, a year on, was the minute bubble. I realized the entire measuring and ordering would take a grand total of ten minutes, and I finally got my ass into gear to do it.

(Guess how long this almighty task *actually* took? Three minutes, 44 seconds. Golly. No wonder I didn't have time.)

9-TO-5ERS WHO DREAM OF EASY STREET

Easy street. It's the fabled place where the extraordinary among us live, while the rest of us slum it in difficult street.

There's a Western obsession with retiring young. We fixate on the corner office but once we get it, we realize it's as much (or more) work, just of a different type. We're still balls to the wall. So we flip our gaze upwards once more. One day we'll get there. To the street of ease. Where we are a person what lunches, with a hard-bodied personal trainer.

I happened upon the phrase 'There is no such thing as easy street' through one of my favourite podcasts, *The One You Feed*. I listened to the episode 'No Easy Street' over and over and over, as it impaled both a fantasy and a frustration of mine.

There is no easy street. Huh. So no wonder I can't get there, no matter how hard I work.

Even if there were, we probably wouldn't want it. We're told that pleasure is in the bumming around, the untempered clicking, the acres of free time, the hiatus from the bore-off ballache of work. But the opposite is true, I've found.

I now know that I don't want easy street, because I have the option to live there, and I choose not to. I've been freelance for nine years now, so I can do as little or as much work as I want (as long as I make rent, bills and the grocery shop, obviously).

And yet, even though I am the architect of my own day, I bet it looks a heckofalot like yours, if you are 9-to-5.

Although I spent a good few years there wearing PJs and no make-up all day (I think because I was suffering from 'dress up and schlepp to work in the big city' PTSD), I have now discovered that my 'this works, I'll do this' routine has become uncannily similar to what I did *before* I was my own boss.

I usually start work at 9am and do eight hours. I turn my phone off while I'm working. I even pay to go to a co-working space five days a week. A few years ago, leisure-wear-clothed me (who had upgraded from PJs) would have been like, 'Are you having a giraffe, why would I choose to go to an office when I have fled that tyranny?!'

But I did a trial and I loved it. 'I get so much more done here!' I said to a staff member. 'It's because if you watch Netlix here, people WILL judge you', she replied.

I found that given my work desk was at home, I never fully switched off from work. Now I *can*. Co-working has given me back that beautiful delineation between work and home. I get that 6pm feeling of leaving the office. And best of all, that Friday feeling of knowing it's all done until Monday.

Oh, and while we're here, the weekend set-up is perfect. Even though I can legitimately do DIY or see my mates all week, I do tend to keep it to the weekend now. Five days on, two off (or four/three when I feel like a long weekend) is the ideal balance of productivity/leisure. Because productivity is pleasure.

Test this out one weekend. Spend Saturday doing sweet FA. Horizontal, watching back-to-back films, ordering takeaway. Then spend Sunday doing the complete opposite. And note your happiness levels at the end of each day. It's a modern myth that kicking back is the square root of happiness. Some lying around at the end of a hard work day is delicious, but all day? Starts to feel profligate.

'People mistakenly think happiness is the absence of negative emotion,' says Dr Korb. 'But if you're always trying to avoid negative emotions, you won't do anything important. The cost of doing something of value is almost *always* hard work. Focusing on the value, rather than the cost, is the key.' We have to get willing to be uncomfortable, he says, rather than trying to steer towards easy street.

Effort is how we build our best possible lives. And the way you know you're doing life right? At times you say, 'I can't do this' and 'this is too much' because THAT means you are living outside of your comfort zone, pushing, striving and growing.

Nothing truly great ever happens in your comfort zone. Nobody grows there.

ODES TO THE ORDINARY

An ode to doing your tax return

It's something we allow to swing over us all year like a guillotine.

It's something that we tell ourselves will take for-ev-er.

We put it off, and procrastinate, and bury ourselves in the duvet of denial. Until the deadline is breathing down our necks and we are forced to do it.

I always tell myself that my tax return is a behemoth of a task that will take me two full days, and thus find other things to put in front of it. 'Ah, brilliant, there's another thing!' *Carefully places it in front of tax return*

But last year, I decided to add up how long the entire process took, from trawling my bank statements, to adding up invoices, to sorting through a small blizzard of receipts that I had carefully filed away by shoving them into a box.

And no, I do not do month-by-month expenses, or earnings, or any of that calculate-as-you-go nonsense. WHO DOES THAT? I don't understand those people.

Anyway, I literally clock-watched the entire procedure of doing a year's worth of earnings and expenses, and do you know how long it took? A measly, underwhelming, what was all the fuss about, six hours. Yep.

If you're like me, and you're just filing as an individual, I bet you'll find the same. When you actually add up the hours, it's not that long. And there is such a sweet satisfaction to be had in filing it early.

We award tax returns more pain in our heads than they actually caused, because much of the pain was created in the guillotine swinging about over us, which was fashioned from the steel of our own procrastination.

I wouldn't say doing your tax return is a joy. I could never go that far. But having *done it* is. It's a delicious, luxuriously ordinary triumph, pressing 'send' on that heinous thing, and we often forget to absorb *how good it feels*.

I WANT TO BE AN 'INFLUENCER'

My nephew recently told me that when he grows up, he's going to be a famous YouTuber, who makes millions from playing video games. I wouldn't say his ambition is an uncommon one, in today's kids. It's a bit like how we all wanted to be ballerinas or firemen.

I have so many friends who follow all of the rules in order to leap-frog from an 'ordinary' amount of followers, into the promised land of an 'extraordinary' amount of acolytes. They hashtag their faces off, they post daily, they do videos of them working out. It's exhausting, and most of all, ill-advised.

It's a safe bet that Instagram influencers spend a lot of time on Instagram, right? I'm willing to wager that the professional 'influencers' spend at least two hours a day on the 'gram, given their propensity to post pictures and videos daily. And a recent study showed that the more time you spend on Instagram, the higher your rates of anxiety and depression.

The 2018 study (which only looked at women, to be fair, aged between 18 and 35), found that 'the frequency of Instagram use is correlated with depressive symptoms, self-esteem, general and physical appearance anxiety, and body dissatisfaction'. Yeesh.

Then there was my favourite headline of 2017:

FACEBOOK 'MAY MAKE YOU MISERABLE', SAYS FACEBOOK
Sky News

Give that headline-writer a gold star.

The study found that liking posts, clicking through to links and updating your status on Facebook leads to a decrease of five to eight per cent in 'self-reported mental health'.

'Today I took 56 selfies'

Imagine the reality of being an 'influencer'. You have to think of inventive ways to advertise a smoothie, which probably makes you feel like a dipstick. 'Yay, smoothie time! Mmmm, I love the kale, spirulina, kimchee and ox hair combo in this bad boy!' Cue: cringe.

You have to move all of your stuff so that it looks like you live in an Anthropologie showroom. You have to do your hair on a daily basis, rather than having hedgerow-hair days, which I am personally very fond of. You can't eat food without taking pictures of it, or doing a demonstration video as to how you made it. People ask you what you did at work today, and your honest reply has to be, 'took 56 selfies of me and my dog'.

Also, Instagram merely compounds the misguided belief that the extraordinary is where the happiness is at. A quick cursory glance down my Instagram will reveal me outside Chichén Itzá, a topless dude rowing me about alligator-infested swamps in Florida, me beside a person-sized display of my books in WHSmith and the marvellous birthday cake my sister-in-law made me.

The way we almost exclusively brag about our extraordinary moments, negates the ordinary loveliness in between. These were all 'extra' days on my Instagram feed, and all very pleasurable indeed, but there was a vast swathe of ordinariness in between that went uncatalogued by Instagram. Thankfully, I lasso them in my gratitudes, but my ordinary moments are invisible on social media.

Givers of repeated experiences

Hold up; aren't we just capturing experiences? And we know now that experiences make us happier than stuff? So, where's the harm in that?

But when I just said 'experiences', I bet you auto-whimsyed yourself atop Machu Picchu, or staring at Petra, right? For all our awareness, we still treasure expensive experiences over ordinary ones. Failing to see that that's just another type of consumerism. The McDonald's in the Louvre is testament to that.

The Starbucks at the foot of an ancient Pyramid triggered the spoof News Thump story headlined 'Big void at centre of Pyramid revealed to be a Starbucks!' 'Scientists made the discovery yesterday,' they wrote, 'after drones they had deployed returned from the inside of the pyramid with a pumpkin spice latte, a mocha frappe and a Danish pastry.'

Buying items that give us repeated pleasurable experiences is where it's at, (rather than an insanely expensive ticket to an 'escape' room experience or the opera) says Professor Lyubomirsky. 'Like a guitar, a picture book, a dress, a camera, cake decorating lessons or running shoes,' she says.

Also, some of the most satisfying 'experiences' can be the most quaint. You don't have to be at Angkor Wat to be having a blast. I had an absolute ball once looking around a lamp museum. And don't even get me started on the 'fries museum', which was a riot. Titchy, quirky tourist attractions are often even more fun.

Capturing it kills it

Some experts even think that capturing it, or manically taking photos for social media, kills our ability to remember it. They call this the 'photo-taking impairment effect'. They discovered this by leading a bunch of students round an art gallery, and noting who photographed what. Afterward, they discovered that the students remembered the paintings they had *merely looked at*, rather than photographed, more vividly.

It makes sense, doesn't it? You can't fully be in the moment if you're obsessed with the angle of a film or photo. It's the dispiriting sight of thousands of phones being held aloft at a gig, videoing the music, rather than the people dancing to it. They have become human selfie sticks, rather than gig goers.

I've done it, of course. Take a picture of me eating waffles in a diner! Take a picture of me underwater with these fish! (Which promptly scares off the fish.) Take a picture of me on this boat pretending to stare off into the distance romantically! (Then analyses photo to see if it's adequate instead of admiring undulating ocean.)

I take four months off social media a year and oh my, do I need it. Before my break, I start to get into that 'Instagram director' headspace of 'What's the point in us hiking up this mountain unless we take 30 pictures of it?' or 'There's a swing in the café! Let's do an Instagram story about it, rather than messing about on it and chatting.'

But, hang on. Whoa there. Looking back at photos often gives me joy. I don't think all photo-taking slays your ability to be in the moment. I love taking and revisiting photos! So, where does the distinction lie?

I think here: if you fully absorb and immerse yourself in something, and then take a photo *to remember the moment*, rather than taking the photo *instead of having the moment*. The 'impairment' comes, I believe, with extensively choreographed shots, faked 'moments', or racing around a gallery and snapping instead of staring.

Whereas spontaneous, quick-fire photos? Let's carry on regardless.

Careful what you wish for

Fame is a dubious ambition. I am far from famous, but these days I get a lot of emails from strangers, or from people I haven't seen for 20 years.

This is because being in the public eye comes with an unanticipated side order. Practically overnight, something shifts, and suddenly lots of people want something from you. I have had dozens of people, who wanted nothing to do with me before my first book was published, sliding from obscurity and wanting to hang.

This means you can never really be sure if they like you for you. I have been asked 'out' on what I thought was a friend date, only to discover that they merely want me as a guest for their podcast. I have gone for a coffee with someone I haven't seen for years, only to discover they just want me to hook them up with my agent.

My feed is filled with the most supersized praise – you've saved my life – I love you – you should get an MBE – which my ego rolls around in like a dog in fox excrement.

But, people also inexplicably think it's appropriate to tag me (make sure she sees!) in posts where they talk about how poorly written or excruciating they found my books to be. I mean, I am sorely tempted to go through their tweets and comment on how excruciating and poorly written *those* are but I don't, because I don't want to become one of the writers who doesn't write any more books because they're too busy arguing with people on Twitter.

I've been trolled by many men, who totally ignore what I've just written and merely appraise my appearance as a 'pump then dump' or a 'five-pinter', despite my being a writer rather than a model. (Even then, it wouldn't be OK.)

Nobody should be subject to the worst things people think about them. And yet, that's what happens once you go public. Being in the public eye is a curious crowd-surf, *smash on our face*, *get picked up by the crowd* type of ride. I'm not sure I'd recommend it for your mental health.

'If you ask me what's harder, being famous or flying to space, I'd say fame is much harder,' said Yi So-Yeon, the first Korean to fly into space. While Winona Ryder once said, 'People come up to you and touch you. That's scary, and they seem to think it's OK to do it. Like you're public property'.

Once you're famous, an influencer, or once you've gone public, it's very hard to reverse that. Many household names would no doubt give their right arm for ordinary obscurity, and for the anonymity of being able to walk down a street unrecognized.

ODES TO THE ORDINARY

An ode to savings

Much like with the driving, I have a unique perspective on savings, given I didn't have any until just recently. And skippydeedoo this feels good, now I understand why most of you people do it! Big earnings may not be the ticket to eternal happines, but small savings do help.

The three in four Brits who do have savings, have on average £4,000, said a survey last year. Having savings has produced an unexpected effect, I've found. Now that I have them, I am more thrifty. Huh.

I have no idea how to explain why. I feel sure the Germans should have an extra-long word to define it. The word 'thrift' is associated with being a cheapskate, but it actually originates from 'condition of thriving' and 'prosperity, savings'.

I now understand how thrifty can feel good. I lived in the seaside town where I now reside on an absolute shoestring in my early twenties and frequently ate 69p pasties or a Snickers bar for lunch. And yet, I recall occasionally getting a £4 taxi back from the station rather than walking the 20 minutes. Flopping into it after a (to be fair) 12-hour day in London.

Now I am appalled by my frivolity! Now I never get that taxi. My town would have to be swallowed by a tornado to convince me to take that taxi.

There's an ordinary joy to be located in doing things like carefully snipping out money-off coupons. Or buying cheap vintage picture frames and then only having to spend a little on having the print mounted. Or taking your own flask of tea rather than paying a morally reprehensible 20× mark-up. Loading up on buy-one-get-one-frees also turns me on.

It's as if I'm a mythical creature who is now guarding a hard-won pot of gold. When there was just a bit of small change scattered around, why bother? Now I am ferocious about protecting what I've painstakingly earned.

A note to those with no savings

Maybe you're not 'terrible with money', like people say, if you're in the quarter of Brits who have no savings. Maybe you just don't earn enough to save.

People have always told me that money burns a hole in my pocket, and when I was drinking, I was indeed a fiscal fuckwit, doing things like frequently tipping over my overdraft limit (and being charged the now outlawed 'unauthorized overdraft fee' of £25) to service my addictions by buying wine and cigarettes.

But since I quit both addictions, there have been times when I thought I was still awful with money, but here's what it was; I was only just earning enough to get by. Sometimes less than enough. Meaning that if a surprise expense hit, even if it was just £50, it resulted in my needing the 'phone a friend' loan lifeline

Back then, I was in a constant state of financial self-loathing, that I never seemed to have enough. But now, I look back and admire how I managed on so little.

The true mark of how good you are with money, is what you do with it once *you have enough*, or more than enough. So, I salute you, skint comrades. I know. Having money means it's easier to be good with it.

VI: ORDINARY BRAINS
AND DOWNTIME

ODES TO THE ORDINARY
An ode to having a run-of-the-mill IQ

We long to be geniuses. To be 'special'. To be carted off to Hogwarts due to unseen magical abilities. (Just me? Err well, this is awkward.)

And yet, when I think rationally about it, I imagine having a high IQ is a bit like being sober in a roomful of batfaced people. Or speaking fluent French in a room of high school French students. Ernest Hemingway clearly agreed, because he wrote: 'Happiness in intelligent people is the rarest thing I know'.

A famous study of extraordinary geniuses was undertaken by a psychologist called Lewis Terman in the 1920s, who searched Californian schools for 1,500 kids who had IQs of 140 and upward. The kids were called 'The Termites' due to his name.

He tracked The Termites throughout their lives. Many of this elite group did go on to do very special things. One wrote *I Love Lucy*. Overall, they earned twice as much as your average bear. Terman wrote of their outstanding achievements:

'Nearly 2,000 scientific and technical papers and articles and some 60 books and monographs in the sciences, literature, arts, and humanities have been published. Patents granted amount to at least 230. Other writings include 33 novels, about 375 short stories, novelettes, and plays; 60 or more essays, critiques, and sketches; and 265 miscellaneous articles on a variety of subjects.'

But many just went for regular jobs. And overall, The Termites' levels of divorce, addiction and suicide were the same as the American average. Their intelligence didn't inoculate them against life's hard knocks.

What's more, many of the Termites were re-interviewed in their eighties and a trend was found. Many reported feeling that they hadn't lived up to lofty expectations set of them when they were kids.

There it is again. The 'high expectations' as the petri dish in which future disappointments are grown. Huh. It seems to be a repetitive lesson being thrust at us, no?

IN DEFENCE OF BEING
AVERAGELY INFORMED

Ordinary news consumption: doesn't really give a flying fuck.

Extraordinary news consumption: mastermind with a keen social conscience.

Consuming an extraordinary amount of news is actively bad for our mental health. We would all, without exception, be more joyful on an ordinary amount of news. But merely saying that makes me feel like people are heaping medieval curses upon my head, and muttering about my being a bad citizen. Our live news feeds mean we can watch devastations and atrocities unfold in real time. We can watch the Notre Dame cathedral smoulder, smoke billow from it, its gorgeous windows crack, its artworks turn to smoke. We watch bombs detonating over and over and over. We watch CCTV footage of people with samurai swords or AK-47s, filmed just before a mass murder.

Watching the daybreak news is essentially like taking a sledgehammer to a hopeful little mole of morning happiness. And not all forms of news are created equally, in terms of our stress response.

'Videos are often better at engaging our attention than reading,' says neuroscientist Dr Korb. 'So, watching something is more likely to activate the limbic system; which makes it feel more visceral. Whereas reading may be more effortful, but it brings the prefrontal cortex online, which helps us be rational.' Reading keeps us objective, essentially.

You are deliberately being agitated

The news is the biggest agitator on the planet. It is written in order to incite the greatest reaction possible, good or bad (usually bad). It is the greatest journalistic minds of our country using their words to pick you up and shake you sadistically, like miniature people trapped a snow-globe.

And yet, we are complicit. We seek out this stress. We hang onto our daily headlines like a news reporter hanging onto a lamppost, while reporting on a hurricane.

Why do we do this? We don't need to do this. Yet the propaganda publishing press that lives in our head, and churns out finger-wagging scolding, tells us that *we do*.

News journalists do, of course, trigger titanic social change. One picture, or one clip, can set globe-changing events into motion. But, much of what is broadcast is sensationalized, exaggerated and alarmist, because that snags higher viewing and reading figures.

'Negative sensationalism in news has been gradually increasing over the past 20–30 years,' writes Professor of Psychology Dr Graham Davey, who has spearheaded studies into the psychological impact of news, and is the author of *The Anxiety Epidemic*.

In 1997, Davey and colleagues conducted a study whereby they showed participants three types of 14-minute news round-ups; positive, negative and neutral. 'As we predicted, those who watched the negative news bulletin all reported being significantly more anxious,' he concluded. More sorrowful too.

The study also showed that those exposed to the negative news tended to then go on to talk about their 'main worry' in life more and catastrophize how it might shake out long-term.

So, in short, the news not only hoiks up our anxiety and depression about the thing we've just seen, but it also makes us more likely to distress our personal life worries, like a dog with a chew toy.

I see this happening constantly. I've just been talking to a four-months-pregnant friend, who told me that the hormones sprinting around her body have resulted in her becoming addicted to checking newspaper headlines. Possibly, this is her body trying to scan the environment for negative things that may harm her baby. And now, her limbic system is freaking out about reports of Iranian boats attempting to besiege a British oil tanker.

Her fears are not irrational; far from it. I mean, how could you *not* worry about something like that? I started worrying about it too, once she told me. And yet, the siege was evaded, and neither of us can do diddly squat about it, anyhow. So our fears are rational, yet largely futile.

The news is not finite anymore

My stepdad sits in front of rolling news day in, day out. I don't know how he sits there, beatific, while politicians hurl word grenades at each other during debates. I can only conclude that he is an unsung spiritual leader who is wasted as a black cab driver in Marston Green, and may well be deified after he dies.

Baby Boomers grew up in an age where news consumption was finite. It was pretty easy to know the news. There was the lunchtime and evening news, at half an hour a pop, and you usually just caught one of them. You only bought one newspaper, rather than attempting to read five online.

These days, the news is utterly indomitable. Apparently web content now doubles between every nine and 24 months. Trying to keep abreast of it is like trying to stay astride a bucking bronco while wearing silk PJs.

And the main emotion we feel when we watch it is: powerlessness. Which has given rise to a host of unusual ways people try to take the power back. Back when Christine Blasey Ford publicly accused supreme court justice nominee Brett Kavanaugh of sexually assaulting her, a group of women did something novel. To deal with the news of Kavanaugh being confirmed into the supreme court, they gathered in a New York bookstore to place a hex on him. The ritual included graveyard dirt, effigies, coffin nails and of course, incantations. In their spell-casting eyes, they were doing something worthwhile to help.

Installing 'medium' news caps

Dr Davey thinks TV schedulers should be held to more rigorous scrutiny, given the psychological fall-out. He and many other experts believe that the impact upon our mental health is such that we should impose limits on our exposure to the news.

They're never going to stop providing a 24/7 looped news cycle, so it's now on us to decide how we consume it.

In my twenties and early thirties, I worked on magazines and newspapers and was over-newsed. I was expected to be informed on everything happening in the world. On some jobs, they expected me to read every Saturday and Sunday newspaper which, lemmetellyou, would have taken all weekend if I had ever actually managed it. BBC News and Sky News were on at all times in the newsroom. Not only that, I was asked to check celebrity gossip blogs every day.

I was stuffed full of anxiety from alarmist news reporting, my specialist subject on any quiz night was the minutiae of celebrity's lives, and I felt horrible about my body thanks to constantly looking at pictures of celebs in bikinis on the Sidebar of Shame.

When I quit drinking, I started questioning everything, including my news intake. Prior to that, I would often buy three newspapers a day, in order to fleece them for feature ideas.

Newly sober, I started noticing that when I consumed too much news, I was mentally constructing a house made of cockroaches in order to survive a nuclear winter. Observing that I grew angry and depressed after a news binge, especially post-Trump inauguration and Brexit vote.

I started digging around in all of the aforementioned evidence that shows that the news can be kindling for anxiety and despair. Why it's addictive. And exploring what the best ways are to get your news. (Listening to the radio apparently lifts people's spirits more than TV.)

I lived abroad for a few months and took the opportunity to take a total sabbatical from the news. As a result, I felt much calmer, more present and less freaked out by people with large backpacks on public transport. My news diet had zero effect on the world, given I have very little influence over it, but it created within me a state of zen.

The entire time, I felt guilty, like I *should* be reading and watching, like I was living in a privileged fairyland, sticking my fingers in my ears going la-la-la-la while people suffered. But then I realized, me knowing about every terrible thing happening in the world does nothing to stop it.

I now swerve all televised news. I'm very careful to keep my 'news diet' wholesome and non-hysterical, I never click on shock news-bait. I never watch gruesome smartphone videos of real-life events. One Saturday and one Sunday newspaper are now my limit of news intake. That's still about four hours of news-reading a week, given it takes me a while to plough through them. As a result, my state of mind is enormously improved.

And yet, given my cap, my finger is not on the immediate pulse, so whenever someone brings up a breaking current affair, I feel as if I'm back at university, haven't done the required reading, and I'm about to be examined on it. It's like one of those dreams where you're in the classroom naked.

The social shaming of news-capping

'Don't you want to know what's going on in the world?' my parents ask me when I dive out of the room during the evening news. They are both news hounds who check headlines several times a day. They then come to me and tell me, 'Did you hear about [insert freak murder]? Isn't it terrible?' And I want to un-know what they just told me.

We have a prejudice against positive psychology, culturally. 'We're told that you only grow through negative experiences, and that which doesn't kill you makes you stronger, and if you're not upset you're not paying close enough attention,' says neuropsychologist Dr Hanson. So far, so gloomy.

This low hum of prejudice is why those who choose to prioritize their own well-being, whether by swerving the news, or saying no to favours they don't have time to do, are stigmatized as la-di-dah rejectionists of real life. You're being selfish, or not looking out for others, or you will no longer be politically active. 'But actually, anxiety and depression make people less generous and less inclined to get engaged politically,' points out Dr Hanson.

It's important to recognize this prejudice against protecting your own well-being, he says. 'Like other forms of implicit bias, such as sexism or racism, it needs to be called out of the corner in order to be dealt with.' It's an elephant in many rooms.

If a current affair is something I can influence, such as in the run-up to an election, then bring it on. If it's something local I can assist with, then come to me. If I was there at the scene, I would of course HELP, but if I can't help, why do I have to watch it unfold?

Sending a donation is much more constructive than knowing the minutiae of what's happened. It's more important to ask how we can help, rather than mindlessly watching, or hitting 'share' and feeling like a social warrior.

The allotment metaphor

The way I now see it is this. I have a corner of ground in a vast allotment. It's enormous, this allotment. And I just need to tend my patch.

I'm in my allotment, and the miles and miles of square plots as far as the eye can see, are other people's gardens. Fire fighters, non-crooked politicians, ocean conservationists, plastic campaigners and charity directors. I can't garden all of their plots, so I'm just going to focus my efforts on mine.

One issue I choose to put in my allotment is this. Rough sleeping has risen by 134 per cent since 2010 in Britain. And our current homeless population is set to double by 2041. It's an inconvenient truth that I can't continue to walk past; our homeless population needs help.

I once asked a woman who runs a homeless shelter what's best to give our unsheltered, and she said that given addiction is often a cause (or consequence) of homelessness, the best thing to give is the ability to buy hot food and drinks, since many well-wishers buy them cold food.

So now, I almost always carry Greggs gift cards loaded up with enough for a couple of meals and drinks, and hand those out instead of cash. The response is always confusion, then delight, given the agency to choose a meal and hot drink. And I feel like it's somehow less humiliating than a cash handout. (If you're abroad, check with local café chains to find out who does pre-loaded pay cards and won't turn the homeless away. Or just take a flask and selection of sandwiches out yourself, if you like the idea.)

In winter, thanks to the homeless shelter woman's advice, I also give out socks and gloves, given she said these are rarely donated at clothes banks; they're just chucked instead. Again, when I hand these out, they're snatched up with relief. There's also 'Next Meal', a website which enables you to direct the homeless to the nearest free food.

What's in your allotment? We can't fix it all simply by *knowing about* it all. There's a fine balance between staying informed and protecting our own mental health. An extraordinary knowledge of current affairs may be socially celebrated, but your brain doesn't like it.

ODES TO THE ORDINARY

An ode to books

Books enable us to travel without moving as much as an inch. I've had a lifelong love affair with them since the age of 11, when I started maxing out my library card. I didn't go abroad until I was 15, and even then it was to a neon-lit strip of a tourist resort, but it didn't matter a whit, because I had already travelled regardless.

I travelled to an alternative England overrun with wolves, via *The Wolves of Willoughby Chase*. I hung out in Sweet Valley High and on the branches of the Magic Faraway Tree. I went through the wardrobe to Narnia. And Louis de Bernières took me to a Greek Island during WWII.

Doomsayers predicted the book's days were numbered, in the early twenty-tens. They said that e-books and the internet would drop-kick print into oblivion. They were, I'm delighted to report, very wrong.

The phoenix rise of print started in 2016, when sales of e-books swan dived by 17 per cent, while physical books finally stopped their alarming plummet, ascending by 8 per cent. 'Could it be, is it, could the book be...back?' people muttered.

Then, in the first half of 2017, it was confirmed by the ker-ching of billions of pounds; with Amazon reporting a book sale surge of 46 per cent. Come 2018, hardback book sales leapfrogged by 31 per cent, while 80 per cent of Brits have recently said they prefer to buy a physical book.

The reasons? Many think it's because of device overwhelm, meaning we reach for actual books instead of e-readers, needing a digital detox. Interestingly, studies have shown that we retain information far better when we read it on physical paper, rather than on a screen. (Even though it's obviously better for the environment to read on a screen.)

It's become cool to post 'shelfies' of your bookshelves/a stack of your current reading list/your nose in a book. Oyster, the so-called 'Netflix for books' folded after just a year. Silent book clubs are A Thing. There's also the fact that books have become strokable and beautiful ornaments, from *Homegoing*, to *H is for Hawk*, to *The Essex Serpent*.

My books are friends that I return to again and again. I crack the spine unapologetically, I turn down corners, I highlight with wild abandon, I write notes in the margins, I lend them to mates. I found that when I read e-books I read more, but enjoyed it less; it felt like snacking, rather than sitting down for a slow luxurious meal.

> 'What an astonishing thing a book is. It's a flat object made from a tree with flexible parts on which are imprinted lots of funny dark squiggles. But one glance at it and you're inside the mind of another person, maybe somebody dead for thousands of years. Across the millennia, an author is speaking clearly and silently inside your head, directly to you. Writing is perhaps the greatest of human inventions, binding together people who never knew each other, citizens of distant epochs. Books break the shackles of time. A book is proof that humans are capable of working magic.'
>
> Carl Sagan, *Cosmos*

ODES TO THE ORDINARY
An ode to whodunnits

Watching a cat-and-mouse murder mystery, while relaxing with dinner-on-a-tray, is one of our favourite ordinary pastimes. Our appetite for psychopathic protagonists is remarkable.

It's why shows like *CSI, The Fall, Luther, Hannibal, Marcella* and *Dexter* are runaway successes. *NCIS* is the world's third most watched show, behind football and bizarrely, the totally unfunny (in my view) *Big Bang Theory*.

I'm in. It's slightly worrying that my viewing of choice almost always involves people getting murdered. But it seems we're not swotting up to become serial killers, say experts. Our urge to watch murder mysteries taps into something primal, natural, normal. It's more because they remind us of roller coasters, and they put us through mental gymnastics, limbering up our brains. 'Serial killers tantalize people much like traffic accidents, train wrecks or natural disasters,' writes Scott Bonn, a criminology professor at Drew University, in a piece for *Time* magazine. He says that witnessing terrible deeds gives us a jolt of adrenaline.

'Adrenaline is a hormone that produces a powerful, stimulating and even addictive effect on the human brain', he continues. 'If you doubt the addictive power of adrenaline, think of the thrill-seeking child who will ride a roller coaster over and over until he or she becomes physically ill.'

Meanwhile, Dr Amanda Ellison, a neuroscientist at Durham University, wrote a piece for *The Telegraph* saying that a Nordic noir box set is an excellent work out for the brain; 'watching a powerful mystery is actually good for you,' she writes. 'That's neuroscientific fact.'

It's all about the twists, the turns, the false leads, the complex spiderweb of characters. 'The best TV crime dramas build suspense over a number of episodes,' according to Dr Ellison. 'They challenge viewers to pay attention to complicated stories, including red herrings, and to remember them from episode to episode.'

'In other words, they provide great stimulation for the brain', she continues, 'which in turn helps keep it healthy, as the human brain needs to be kept active. In fact, when you deprive it of stimulation it reacts very badly.'

'The more you tax your brain, the sharper it becomes,' Dr Ellison concludes. 'And when you watch complex TV drama, you really tax it.'

A whodunnit from the sofa is, I conclude, a decadently ordinary evening's entertainment which is basically the equivalent of a Sudoku puzzle. What's not to like about that?

REDISCOVERING NINETIES AVAILABILITY

The smartphone revolution has snuck into our lives, bit by megabit, slunk up behind us and shoved us into a bear-trap. A bear-trap of extraordinary connectivity. We have lost the beauty of ordinary availability, given we now all have devices that clamp us into *always being on*.

Here's how it was in the nineties:

Person A phones person B's house phone.

Person B is out – or doesn't feel like answering.

Person A does not know which one it is.

Person A leaves a message.

Person B phones them back the next day, or whenever they twattin' well feel like it, because person A does not own person B.

You may have detected a note of raging against the machine in my tone, a longing for us to go back to the halcyon days when our expectations of each other were much lower. You're not wrong.

See, we've been tricked into a noughties nightmare, a digital predicament, whereby that 24–48 hour totally acceptable get-back-to-you window has shrunk.

Way back when, you had a good two weeks to call Aunt Margaret and thank her for her card, a month to pay, six weeks to respond to a penpal. Then emails came along and, suddenly, the time-windows shortened. Responses became expected more quickly, but only within a week. Then the vice tightened to a few days.

Then text messages tapped and bleeped their way into our existence, and all of a sudden, you need to pay bills instantly or they incessantly message you about late payment charges, or friends and family follow up with 'Hello?'s within a few hours.

This stranglehold, this feeling that a convenience-enhancer has become a time-burglar, is why a US study found that the mobile phone has become the invention we hate most, yet feel we can't live without (beating the alarm clock and hoover). It's why it's become a status symbol, a hipster version of sticking it to The Man, a rejection of the lemming march, to now carry a good ol' Nokia.

Tarantino famously has a 'no mobile phones' policy on set, and personally eschews all text and email. If you want to contact him, you have to phone his home phone and leave a message on an answering machine. Retro!

Our phones are sticky

The world's most cunning fox-like tech minds are currently hard at work making their apps and phones evermore 'sticky', which is tech-bro speak for 'frickin' addictive'.

Previously a design ethicist at Google, Tristan Harris is one of many ex-tech-colluders that have turned whistleblower after fleeing their digital hosts. In his 2017 Ted talk *How a handful of tech companies control billions of minds every day*, he revealed, 'every news site, TED, elections, politicians, games, even meditation apps have to compete for one thing, which is our attention, and there's only so much of it. And the best way to get people's attention is to know how someone's mind works. And there's a whole bunch of persuasive techniques that I learned in college, at a lab called the Persuasive Technology Lab, to get people's attention'.

Persuasive technology is wily. 'Autoplay' functions on Netflix, Facebook and YouTube, which hook you into another video or episode without even waiting for you to press play. Snapchat's 'Snapstreaks' function, where ~~teenagers~~ users get rewarded for communicating with each other for a block of days in a row, and thus don't want to lose their streak.

Harris says the parents think, 'Oh, they're just using Snapchat the way we used to gossip on the telephone. It's probably OK. Well, what this misses,' he points out, 'is that in the 1970s, when you were just gossiping on the telephone, there wasn't a hundred engineers on the other side of the screen who knew exactly how your psychology worked and orchestrated you into a double bind with each other'. Cue a generation of extremely sleep-starved teens – and adults.

In short, we're being manipulated by terrifically clever people into doing things we don't necessarily want – or need – to do. 'If you see a notification, it schedules you to have thoughts that maybe you didn't intend to have,' adds Harris.

Feeling outraged by this digital mind control? A-ha, therein lies another way they pull on your emotional puppet-strings. Harris reveals that outrage is often harnessed by these tech giants too, whereby they waggle things they know will incite you, having monitored your browsing history and thus gained access to your beliefs. 'Click-hate', if you will. 'And because this is profitable, it's only going to get worse,' he warns.

Screen bans in Silicon Valley

It's well known that many Silicon Valley parents now restrict their children's use of screens – or outright ban it – for this very reason.

A former executive assistant at Facebook, Athena Chavarrian (who still works for Mark Zuckerberg in his philanthropic pursuits), is a total rejectionist of pre-high school phones. 'I am convinced the devil lives in our phones and is wreaking havoc on our children,' she told *The New York Times*.

In the same *New York Times* piece, the former editor of *Wired* and father-of-five, Chris Anderson, said, 'On the scale between candy and crack cocaine, it's closer to crack cocaine'.

Steve Jobs didn't let his kids near iPads; Bill Gates banned phones until high school (his wife Melinda wished they'd waited longer) and takes a week-long tech break himself every six months; while the CEO of Apple, Tim Cook, has been quoted saying he doesn't allow his nephew to use social media.

Why? They know how addictive it is.

Phones are the new cocaine

We're on the hedonic treadmill while we're on our phones, too. Psychotherapist and author of *The Phone Addiction Workbook*, Hilda Burke, compares 'like' addiction to cocaine use. When you very first joined Instagram or Facebook, 10 likes was enough; then 50 was your new ideal buzz; and on and on. It unfolds much in the same way an addiction takes hold, meaning the cocaine user habituates over time, and thus needs fatter lines to reach their desired high. Needing more likes is the same process. 'You post more, share more, sacrifice more of your personal time and space to get the same hit,' she says.

Our reliance has become so unreal that Burke discovered that even massage therapists now bemoan having to prise phones out of their clients' hands. 'If we cannot bear to be separated from our smartphones for a 50-minute relaxation treatment, it's clear that we have an extremely dysfunctional relationship with our devices,' she says.

I reminisce about how plane journeys used to be such a welcome Wi-Fi-free zone, and now *even there* we can access social media, which feels like an invasion of a sacred space. 'I think the same,' says Burke. 'It's only inhibited by the fact you have to pay for it. I dread the day it becomes free.'

'I do think we've now reached "peak phone"', Burke adds. 'Now everyone knows the damaging repercussions of overuse. Ten years ago when iPhones were shiny and new, if somebody had suggested that you limit your time on it, you would have been like "Why?! It's amazing!" We didn't know, until recently.'

'The awakening we're undergoing is much the same as how we would have regarded cocaine when it was first imported to the UK,' she says, 'before the dark side started to manifest, and it was banned in 1920.' If you'd asked an 1890s person what they thought of cocaine, it would have been much the same as what a 2007 person thought of manic phone use. 'I love it! Why stop?'

Our phones are snitches

Another way they make phones supremely sticky, is by turning them into snitches. Curtain twitchers, that are like 'I can see her, she's there!' Apps like WhatsApp, Twitter and Instagram know full well that their snide little 'seen' or 'online' telltales, or that little blue dot, is like app Velcro.

They have thrown us under the bus, and made it so that the sender of the message can see when we're there. There's no hiding. There's no 'I only just read it' subterfuge. They've whipped that deniability away, while rubbing their hands together with glee.

It's now impossible to swoop in and scoop up your messages without being spotted, which means that we spend far more time 'online' once we're in, since it seems rude to ignore a person 'typing...' to you in real time. We're far more likely to concede and go 'typing...' back. And then the other person feels the sticky social construct too, so they are 'typing...' back. And repeat.

Meaning you both spend 20 more minutes online than you actually intended to, because of their sneaky social obligation glue.

Burke pulls me on this, saying it's not the app to blame, it's my response to it. Ah, shucks. I'd love to blame the app. 'Feeling beholden by the "seen" or "online" function is actually a sign you're probably prone to codependence and people-pleasing,' says Burke. 'If you're placing meeting another's needs over eating your sandwich, that behaviour will play out in other areas of your life too.' Ummm. She may have a point.

Still, I don't see how 'seen' or 'online' or 'read' is socially helpful or necessary. It has never felt helpful or necessary to me. The only thing it has ever done is served as a boot in the behind when someone ignores me, or swipes offline as soon as they see my message; or as a pain in the proverbial, when I'm trying to dodge someone and they can SEE ME.

And they're eradicating ways of turning this guilt-tripping gubbins off. You used to be able to switch off the 'online' function in WhatsApp. Now you can't. I have, of course, turned the double blue-ticking thing off, which tells everyone when you have read a message. (One friend literally asked me to turn it back on 'just for her', because it made her feel 'unimportant' that she could no longer see when I had read her messages. I said no, obviously.)

Instagram has now made it impossible to turn off your DMs; Twitter too, if you follow them back. Which means that strangers can slide into your message requests at any time they choose.

Our 'always on' expectations of each other have created a work/social landscape whereby people feel entitled to huff 'You there?' if you don't respond to their text. (Your phone told tales on you to their phone, that you read that text 3.5 hours ago.)

Work contacts passive aggressively re-name emails 'Did you see this?' and re-send them, two days on, as if you have nothing better to do than craft an elegant reply to their unsolicited request for you to work for free.

Rebelling against it being 'rude not to reply'

I don't remember ever signing up for this. Do you? And I think we need to rebel against it, until it gets even worse, and WhatsApp, I dunno, hack into your camera and starting sending videos of you ignoring messages to the ignored.

But the resistance is building, and ironically, it's mostly mobilizing on socials.

As Holly Whitaker, the founder of an addiction company called Tempest, says on Instagram: 'We've been severely conditioned to believe that social media is necessary, or even that a message that lands in our inbox, SMS, voicemail – whatever – is a contract we've already signed.'

'We are always on,' she continues. 'I can't and won't live that way. There are people whose entire jobs are to keep us coming back to a bottomless pit of distraction from real life, real connection, real work…I don't respond to most messages because I can't, and I don't tie up my worth in my timely responses. I do what I can and don't beat the shit out of myself for dropping the ball or being unreachable.'

This 'it's rude not to reply!' was drummed into us (or me, at least, maybe you relate) back in the mists of time when we only got about 20 emails a week and 10 people texting us a week, maximum.

Many of us now get hundreds of emails a day, and dozens of texts a day. I don't know about you, but given I was raised to reply quickly, these messages bleep in my subconscious, much like an oven timer, until I turn them off by answering them.

By holding each other to this impossible 'you no reply, you rude' standard, we are colluding with the tech titans. Let's give each other permission not to reply sometimes. Rather than holding the accusation of rudeness over one another like a giant wagging foam finger.

A friend recently said to me, 'remember what your job is', when I talked about my indomitable social media inboxes. Sometimes my options are: be 'rude' and do my job, or be polite and not do my job. A lot of days, actually, those are my options. And I have to remember what my job is: writing.

My favourite people these days are those who send thoughtful little rainbows of 'thinking of you' or 'I saw this dog and knew you'd like it' into the ether, without expecting a reply as standard.

Everyone has a million things to do that we know nothing about. This 'it's rude!' narrative is fuelling the madness whereby we check our phones, one study found, on average 150 times a day.

We should reject the 'always reachable' modern anathema. It's like those infuriating dishwashers or washing machines that bleep at you infernally, incessantly, until you empty them. Our devices have begun to control us. We're letting them.

(Some machines are more polite though. I am dogsitting in a house with a washing machine that plays a little ditty every time it finishes a cycle; and then sits in silent anticipation, in the manner of Kate Winslet reclining on that chaise longue in *Titanic*.)

My nineties availability mission commences

The rock bottom for me was this. I went on holiday recently and literally wanted to leave my phone behind. That's how much I'd grown to hate it. But then I realized that it's my music library, my camera, my alarm clock, my online banking device...

As a compromise, I took it with me, but locked it in a safe. I only turned it on five times in ten days. And I felt my shoulders drop about ten inches. I had reclaimed the ordinary phone-checking levels that I had in the nineties.

But when I got home, my usage shot back up to a terrifying, extraordinary average of four hours on it per day. So, I embarked upon a 360 overhaul of my phone habits.

To prepare, I picked up *The Phone Addiction Workbook* by psychotherapist

Hilda Burke and was gobsmacked by what I read. A 2017 study of over 4,000 people found that 66 per cent of Brits check our phones *during the night*. What's more, when smartphone users were given the Sophie's choice of either their phone or sex, a third picked their phone.

Here's what I did, and how it went.

1. Starving the checking addiction

A poll of Americans found that their first thought is their phone, then coffee, then their partner (if they have one).

I relate. I wake up and my brain yells, 'PHONE. WHERE PHONE?' shortly followed by 'COFFEE. WHERE COFFEE?' As someone who was previously addicted to alcohol, I am well aware that when my brain barks orders at me, it's an addiction. It's precisely the same neuroscientific process as when my brain used to growl 'DRINK' at me like Father Jack. And like any addiction, I now know that the only way to shrink it – and weaken it – is to starve it.

The more you check your phone, the more you want to check your phone, says Dr Korb. 'The more we repeat an action and it's rewarded by a dopamine signal, the more likely we are to do it again. Over time, the enjoyable dopamine response decreases because we become habituated to it, but we've already created a habit in the dorsal striatum.' Otherwise known as the 'habit centre' of the brain.

Ironically, when we attempt to *not check our phone*, it creates a mini stress – which gives us more of a dopamine reward once we cave. 'The idea of checking your phone creates a stress and uncertainty in your brain,' says Dr Korb. 'And the way we reduce that is to check our phones. We check it not because we're particularly interested in the information inside, but because of the stress of *not checking it*.'

I start paying attention to what my body does when I hear the call of the phone-checking gremlin. 'Just check, just check, just check,' it chants. My heartbeat quickens, in a cascade of both anticipated pleasure (what treats await!) and anxiety (what threats await!) given the newfound social/work blur.

Morning checking is a particularly tricky badger. Now that our work emails live in our phones, by prodding it into life 45 seconds after we've woken up, we are literally *choosing to be at work 45 seconds after we've woken up*. Bonkers.

It's like pressing a button and – plunk! – tipping ourselves from the bed onto a slide that whooshes us directly to our office chairs, as if in some *Black Mirror* version of a tech company's HQ.

2. Slinging my phone in a drawer for 22 hours a day

See phone, look at phone. I discover from my research that placing an obstacle between me and the phone, will make me less likely to check the phone. My phone-addicted gremlin tries numerous tactics to try and get me to turn my phone back on. 'Here's a really weird cucumber, I need to take a picture of it and WhatsApp it to my cousin who hates cucumbers!' I discovered this; the less you touch your phone, the less you have to do when you touch your phone. Only having my phone on for two hours a day feels heavenly.

3. Using my screensaver as a reminder

We lose hours, days of time down rabbitholes of mindless scrolling, and often find ourselves saying, 'I wish I had more time to.' As a wake-up call, Hilda Burke recommends that we use a picture of us doing the thing we wish we had more time to do, on the lock screen of our phone. Us painting, cuddling our kids, doing a handstand on a beach; whatever. Mine is actually reading, given I think I probably read about twice as many books pre-smartphone, so I try it. It works. But I wonder how long it will work for. 'Once you've achieved what you set out to do, whether that was walking your dog twice a day rather than just once, change the picture,' she suggests.

4. Deleting Facebook

I then attempt to delete Facebook, having seen the Danish Happiness Research Institute study which found that daily users who quit Facebook for a week became 55 per cent less stressed out.

However, they don't make it easy to go AWOL. Trying to extricate myself made me 55 per cent *more* stressed out.

Facebook keeps you hooked by darkly announcing that they will delete your messages and photos forevermore if you leave. The prospect of losing upwards of 4,000 photos gave me pause. My finger hovers, startled. They give you a 'Download' option, but I don't trust this, I suspect it probably comes with a caveat whereby they can access all your data (totally unsubstantiated speculation), so the alternative was to go through 4,000 tagged photos and save every blinking one. I investigated whether I could just 'hide' my profile, but no.

Deleting Messenger was near impossible, so cue: a couple of upset relatives being upset that I hadn't replied to messages I hadn't even seen. In the end, I had to reactivate Facebook (they give you a cooling-off period) and get a degree in Messenger to figure out how to delete it. But I got there, and jeez, did it feel glorious to hoist that social media to-do overboard.

5. Remembering that I own myself

As already mentioned, messages tug at my sleeve like a child in a supermarket. I attend to the child's request, rather than my own needs.

Whatever your cause of digital overwhelm, I think we've all forgotten this. That we own ourselves. That our time belongs to us. Not other people. And this goes beyond emails. We limp on in friendships that would have ended years ago had they been romantic entanglements, 'because I've been friends with her for *years*'.

We pick up when people call, even when we don't want to. We sit there with a full basket o' fishes each morning and give away every single one, until we have none left for ourselves.

6. No longer allowing my phone to burgle my sleep dust

Phones are not only time bandits, they are also sleep stealers. Looking at a phone after 9pm is like opening a window for a cat-soft burglar to creep in and suck all of the precious sleep dust out of your house.

Prior to this overhaul, I used to drift off to sleep about midnight or 1am. And wake up between 7am and 8am, so only scoring about seven hours' sleep.

Many of my friends are now wearing blue-light blocking glasses in the evening, buying into claims that it means devices don't affect your circadian rhythms as much, but I wonder if these just give us carte blanche to continue looking at screens right up until bedtime. Like a 'detox' liver-cleansing pill which means we feel able to drink more, or feeling like a 'diet' soft drink is utterly innocuous.

'That's a really good point,' says Burke. 'These glasses are brilliant for a computer-based shift worker, but it's far better for the rest of us to just switch our screens off an hour or two before bed. Because it's not just about the blue light; what you're actually viewing is also stimulating.'

Most nights, I now turn my phone off at 8pm. Which means I start feeling seriously sleepy at 10.30pm – and thus get more shuteye.

7. I stopped being a dickhead at dinner

An American friend told me they have a game called 'Don't be a dickhead at dinner' which involves everyone placing their phone into the centre of the table. The first to absent-mindedly reach for their phone pays for the entire meal. I now pretend to play this, to stop myself from giving my friends the message 'what's in my phone is more important than you'.

8. Logging out of my emails once the day is done

I have an email app, like most of us do, which automatically downloads all my emails to my phone. Handy. But it also means that I frequently read work emails long after my day is done, given the come-hither little red notification blob.

I started putting an obstacle between myself and this too. Do I really need to read Gmails at 10pm? No. So I log out of it after work now (keeping the app, just signing out).

I also deleted my Twitter and Instagram apps, given I frequently get work emails on those mediums too. Given social media is no longer 'leisure only', I now treat them like work, and access them on my MacBook. Which means I look at them, at most, twice a day, rather than 27 times a day. Which feels sensational.

9. No longer feeding the trolls

Another thing that phones bring into our living rooms, our bedrooms, our bathtubs is: trolls. Those who spend their free time hunting for people to disagree with, or tear down. As the Buddha said, 'Those attached to perception and views, roam the world offending people.'

I now have a 'don't feed the trolls' zero tolerance strategy. The moment someone trolls me, they get blocked. I'm always interested in healthy debate, but mud-slinging carries no interest to me whatsoever. The 'block' button is beautifully empowering. And highly unlikely to carry any blowback, I've found. You don't know them, so why do they need access to you?

Bad reviews of the acoustic version

Some people won't like this unplugged version of you, just as some people didn't like *Nirvana Unplugged* (and those people are, quite simply, wrong). You can't please all of the people all of the time, as the bumper sticker parrots. And as the woke cliché now goes, those who don't like your new-found boundaries, are always the ones who benefitted from you having none. The ones who won't like your 'ordinary availability' downgrade, will be the ones who liked your 'extraordinary reachability'.

They're still spending their evenings staring at and prodding their phone, waiting for something extraordinary to happen. (Barack followed me back! What d'you think the chances are that he does his own social media?), or for a life-changing work email, or for that tall drink o' water to reciprocate on Bumble.

They're wishing, waiting, anticipating rather than living in their delightfully ordinary evening, and if you've bailed on the phone deal, that's one less person for them to bounce off. Meanwhile, you're off having a rad nineties-style evening of dinner, telly and reading. Their evening is whack, as they're waiting for their phones to chirrup and make 'em happy.

But mostly, people won't care. Or notice. I thought my family and friends would kick up a fuss about my new 8pm phone exile but so far, nobody has excommunicated me, I haven't woken up to ONE message saying, 'Where the hell are you?! Why can't I reach you?!' so that boundary was a surprising doddle and has improved my life galactic amounts.

Not having your phone makes you smarter

Not only can detaching from your phone allow you to e-x-h-a-l-e, it could also make you smarter. The mere presence of your device can clobber your cognitive capacity, said a study from The University of Texas neatly named 'Brain Drain: The mere presence of one's own smartphone reduces available cognitive capacity'.

They took 800 people and asked all of them to switch their phone to silent, and then place it either on the desk, in a bag or in another room. They then gave the people a series of cognitive tests, and discovered that those who had their phone stowed in a separate room had a sharper brain.

Assistant Professor Adrian Ward, one of the leaders of the study, said it's the effort of *not thinking* about your phone that provides the brain drain. 'Your conscious mind isn't thinking about your smartphone, but that process – the process of requiring yourself to not think about something – uses up some of your limited cognitive resources. It's a brain drain.'

This has been backed up by a ream of studies, one by the University of California, Irvine, which found that an interruption (such as a phone call, or a message popping up on our screen in a notification box) takes a sloth-like average of 23 minutes and 15 seconds to recover from. And imagine how many digital interruptions we encounter each day?

Another study commissioned by *The New York Times* discovered that even the mere *threat of interruption* creates the same dumbing-down. They found that, compared to a control group, both the 'Interrupted' and 'On High Alert' (who had been told beforehand to expect an interruption) group got 20 per cent less on a test, than those who were uninterrupted and didn't expect an interruption.

It's no wonder that our gadgets will eventually become our Overlords, given their very presence dumbs us down. It's the perfect crime, in a way. We invented them, then they make us less smart, by bleeping and buzzing and hopping about in our immediate vicinity, and meanwhile they plot our ultimate destruction while we're taking 23 minutes to recover from the phone ringing. Touché, gadgets! The only way we can fight back and stop the Robot Revolution is to turn. the. blighters off. That's our power: the off button.

Gizmo mania

My stepdad has an itchy trigger finger for gadgets. Long ago, he realized that he was going to get a hard time from Mum about buying things like drones and digital cameras, but if he combined her mania for a gleaming just-so house with his technophilia, he was onto a winner.

As a result, they now have a leaf blower, an electric window washer, remote-controlled blinds, an automatic handwash dispenser, a tennis bat that electrocutes insects (sorry Buddhists) and an industrial vacuum which has *gears*, and can also shampoo the carpets – and probably make you a coffee.

In my parents' house, you can no longer open the front door unless your thumb print is stored in the system, and you can no longer turn on the lights unless you know the specific commands, such as, 'Alexa, turn on Savannah Sunset'.

I have dystopian visions of a glitching, cackling Alexa plunging me into darkness, not allowing my stepdad entry and putting Metallica on full-blast as she runs every device in the kitchen simultanously. I don't trust her.

Ten years on, maybe our Maidbot will hold us hostage and make us do all of the hoovering, while she kicks back, flirts with Robocop via telepathic text message, bitches about Siri and drinks the hoover's coffee.

I reckon it's those semi-Luddites among us, those with very ordinary tech, who will survive Alexa-geddon. Those whose iPhone is always three versions behind, whose Siri is turned off, whose TV is only averagely smart, and who have honest-to-goodness keys rather than Bluetooth entry to their home.

I think the ordinary-techs will be the guardians of the last bastion of the human race. Our slight suspicion of 'updates' – our tight wallets – will save us.

Controlling them, rather than vice versa

And yet, none of us would wish to go backwards, would we, really. To a time of candlelight and three-day-long horse-and-carriage rides, or hand-washing clothes, or piles of cassette tapes and no 'shuffle' option, or having to choose a partner from the three singles in your immediate vicinity, or dying of things we can now cure like a snap.

Advancements are astounding, but they also threaten to swallow us up, if we don't become the boss of them, much like *Terminator*, or *I Am Mother*, or *Ex Machina*, or the other hundred-plus cautionary fictional tales.

Let's just send each other messages. And then do other things. That person will reply when they have time, or feel like it. The stranglehold of 'seen' is something making us all develop smartphone claws, digital hunch backs, 'text neck' and overly pronounced thumbs. (I caught myself trying to pinch and enlarge a picture in a magazine recently.)

We shouldn't feel guilty about not being available 24/7. Or be afraid to turn the blue ticks off. Or balk to tell our friends and family, 'I am now not contactable after 9pm and before 10am. If you need me, call before 9pm.'

'But what if there's an emergency!' I hear you cry. Unless you have kids, or an aged parent who lives alone, it is highly unlikely you will be the primary source of immediate aid.

You can always get a burner phone and only give those 'potential emergency' people that number. People will think you're a drug dealer, but just roll with it.

We are desperately missing the downtime our brains need, and used to get, before mobile phones. What was intended as a convenience has wound up controlling us. Have we learnt nothing from *Frankenstein*?

The joy of backsliding to ordinary, retro availability is something I cannot recommend enough.

> 'Do we need the internet in our pockets at all times? Do we need it resting by our pillows at night? Do our seven-year-olds need phones? Do we wish to pass down our own dependency and obsession? It all has to be thought through. We can't just let the tech companies decide for us.'
>
> Zadie Smith, writing in the *Guardian*

ODES TO THE ORDINARY
An ode to learning how to bake a cake

If you're feeling low, uninspired, bleurgh, the absolute best thing you can do is learn how to do something new.

Neuroscientists at the University of Southern California conducted a study, headed by Professor Irving Biederman, that showed the brain gets a fix from learning something new. 'The "click" of comprehension triggers a biochemical cascade that rewards the train with a shot of natural opium-like substances,' said Beiderman.

Some things I have learnt to do that have given me this learning rush:

- How to decorate my very ordinary rented bathroom in Moroccan-esque tile stickers that everyone thinks are real.

- How to breathe on both sides during front crawl.

- How to make peanut butter cookies (they were totally inedible and received the reaction 'are those onion bhajis?' but the creation of them still, inexplicably, made me happy).

- How to 'fall correctly' out of a handstand. Because I need to know how to fall. (I do it a lot.)

But it goes far deeper than tile stickers or bhaji-cookies.

Learning is about personal reinvention. 'Women and men learn that through learning they can make and remake themselves', said the great philosopher and educator Paulo Freire.

THE DIMINISHING RETURNS OF TV

Somewhere along the way, I internalized the belief that 'ultimate relaxation' was to be found in the shape of lying horizontal and watching TV. This meant that I would rush through my walk home from the station, rush through exercise and rush through cooking (all three perfectly relaxing things in themselves) in order to get to the pay-off.

We often 'rush to relax'. It's the parent racing through the bedtime story in order to watch *Grey's Anatomy*, or the yogi who jumps up from Shavasana and then yomps their way home, mat slung over their shoulder like a bayonet, undoing all that loving-kindness zen, in order to reach their premium relaxation time.

And yet, TV has diminishing returns, because of hedonic adaptation. The first episode feels luxurious, the second nice, and by the third we've started hating ourselves for allowing another screen to consume our evening.

It's the same with chocolate, sex, alcohol. We binge and wind up feeling wretched. We think, that episode relaxed me! I enjoyed that! So imagine what another, and another, and another will do. Failing to remember the rule of diminishing returns.

Tellingly, researchers have found that those who cap their TV watching at a maximum of two hours per day, live around a year-and-a-half longer overall. More than 14 hours of TV a week is linked to a higher BMI and more depression. And yet, two-thirds of us (at least, say studies) watch *more than* two hours of telly a day. We sit there, powerless to resist, as our TV takes us to the next episode – and the next.

There is convincing research that shows we'd be better going back to the retro way of an episode a week, says Professor Lyubomirsky. 'Rationing out our favourite shows week by week, given the first episode we watch is the high point in any one session.'

Putting the adult in charge

This is the conversation in my brain, whenever I want to watch TV.

Teenage brain: 'I just want to sit and watch *Stranger Things* all day, this is SO NOT FAIR.'

Adult brain: 'You know that when you actually sit and watch three hours of TV it does not make you happy.'

Kid brain: 'Where's my pony? Want pony.'

Putting our adult selves in charge of TV consumption is much like how Cookie Monster evolves in the later episodes of *Sesame Street*. We were used to seeing him demolish piles of cookies without a moment's restraint, crumbs flying.

But in an effort to encourage self-control in children, Cookie Monster changes. He learns to interrupt his 'see cookie, eat cookie' ways by using various devices; pretending the cookie is a yo-yo, sniffing a smelly boot and so on. Eventually, he is successful.

Cookie Monster was right to interrupt the grab; science says this works. I tell neuroscientist Dr Korb that I have started putting the remote control in a drawer, which appears to help me 'interrupt' the habit. 'That's a great idea,' he says. 'Then you can't just mindlessly reach for it.'

'Me want it (but me wait)' became Cookie's theme tune. 'When me lose control, when me on the brink, need to just calm down, me need to stop and think. Me need control me self, yeah that's the way to live. And then me functioning like an EXECUTIVE,' sings Cookie Monster.

As a result of his new-found restraint, Cookie Monster gains entry to the Cookie Connoisseurs Club, thus his temperance was rewarded with prestige. Amazing.

I think of Cookie Monster often. Me want it. But me wait.

ODES TO THE ORDINARY
An ode to boredom

I currently have 59 podcasts log-jammed in my phone, waiting to be listened to. There are 11 documentaries perched smugly in my watchlist, wagging their fingers at me. We are entangled in the net of too much to do, see, read, listen to.

I honestly don't think I've felt bored since 2004, when I obtained constant access to the internet at home. There's always something to do, read, listen to, watch. So today's kids probably rarely feel bored in today's infinite-tainment landscape.

As a child, I spent days deep in the stacks of the library, but at least it was achievable to read all of the local library. It's now impossible for mastery of information to be attained. It's like being in a neverending library, which sounds like a dream, but is more of a dystopian nightmare.

Boredom births imagination. A blank canvas is required for creation. You devise a game with a stick and a ball. Or you learn to be a boss on Spirograph, or at 'walking the dog' on the yo-yo. Or, you make a bush and a garden gnome family into a kingdom.

Screens have replaced the playground of the great outdoors, tragically. Three-quarters of British children spend less time outside than prison inmates do, said a 2016 study by Natural England. The average child spends twice as long playing on a screen, than they do outside. One in nine has not been to a park, beach, forest or similar in the past year.

Obviously, fears around childhood safety are partially driving this. In the eighties, when I was raised, kids were often ushered outside at 2pm and told to be back in time for dinner.

I spent great swathes of time throwing a football at a kerb ('kerby'), trying to catch sticklebacks with my fingers in streams, building 'houses' out of fallen branches and bombing up and down hills on my BMX, entirely unsupervised, from age ten onwards.

Our ancestors' kids played outside all day long, just like this. 'Instead of sitting in front of PlayStations and Xboxes, hunter-gatherer children played collaborative games that mimicked the activities they would perform when mature adults,' says Professor Cregan-Reid. 'They played at building shelters, war, climbing and hunting.'

It seems to me that today's kids could do with being bored a lot more. And definitely being outdoors a lot more. As could we. We're not prison inmates. So let's stop acting like it.

ON MEDIOCRE YET
EXQUISITE CREATIVITY

There seems to be three myths that abound about creativity.

a) That talent is 'natural' and lives within the magically anointed.
b) That you need to wait for inspiration to strike, as if a butterfly lands upon you.
c) That in order to call yourself 'a song writer', or 'a playwright', or 'a dancer', you need to have made some swag from your work.

None of this is true.

What is true, is this:

1. Creatives have to work goshdang hard to learn their craft, mostly by observing and learning from those creatives who have blazed the same trails.

2. Inspiration does not alight upon you, you seize it. Also, deadlines are not napalm for creativity, as many believe, they are just a necessary part of the process, otherwise you could tinker for-ev-ah. And more tinkering, does not necessarily a better creation make.

3. If you pick up a pen, or a paintbrush, or bust out a running man, you too are a writer, artist, or dancer.

Creativity is also not about whether others appreciate your work, or buy it, or clap, or anything. It's about how it makes you feel. And with that in mind, here are my creativity hacks:

1. Mediocre creativity is just as powerful
Human beings are meant to be creative, and it's more about how the creating switches on a lantern inside of you, rather than assembling something that others admire, that they 'ooh' and 'aah' at like a fireworks display. Even if the music's so bad that it kills every insect within a 60-foot radius stone dead; compose it if it makes you happy. Even if your art is more likely to end up in a tip than on a gallery wall; paint it, if doing so makes you feel still-water calm.

I've said this before, but when I write, it's like I've tipped a jumbled box of jigsaw pieces onto the page and assembled it into a recognizable picture. Writing is how I make sense of who I am, and what I think. Drawing is how my friend Rachel achieves this joined-up satisfaction between her brain and fingers. While other friends make rooms beautiful, or strum on a banjo, or knit, or customize vintage clothes, or create colourful salads.

There is a tendency to feel paralysed by the fear of creating something imperfect. Something 'ordinary'. Nobody has to see this. Nobody but you. You simply need to start. You have all of the time in the world to play with it, shape it, re-do it, scrap parts of it; for now, just *do something*.

2. Chase it with a club
Inspiration is something you chase, not something that alights upon you like a bird. American novelist Jack London once wrote, 'Don't loaf and invite inspiration; light out after it with a club, and if you don't get it you will nonetheless get something that looks remarkably like it.'

As a writer, if I waited until the mood struck me, I'd be waiting forever. Thankfully, legends agree. 'A self-respecting artist must not fold his hands on the pretext that he is not in the mood,' said Tchaichovsky.

While Maya Angelou said, 'What I try to do is write. I may write for two weeks "the cat sat on the mat, that is that, not a rat", you know. And it might be just the most boring and awful stuff. But I try. When I'm writing, I write. And then it's as if the muse is convinced that I'm serious and says, "Okay. Okay. I'll come."'

If you do put yourself out there, you inevitably open yourself up to scrutiny. People trying to bodyslam your whimsy and drag you back down to earth. But, in the words of the inimitable Cher, 'Until you're ready to look foolish, you'll never have the possibility of being great'.

3. Creative cups are never full
I know people who place themselves into a creativity vacuum when writing a book, or a song, or when painting. For fear of being influenced by others. But, as the unoriginal cliché goes, originality does not exist anymore, so just go with it.

Being a writer and not reading is like being someone who wants to get warm, yet refuses to sit next to a fire. Sitting at the hearth of others' writing gets you hot-cheeked and warm-blooded. It un-freezes your fingers.

Allow yourself to regard others' great works and observe exactly how they did it, so that you can learn from it. Fashion designer Rick Owens once revealed that he finessed his pattern-cutting skills by making Versace knock-offs.

4. You can move beyond a block

Creativity works better when you move, I've found. Charles Darwin knew it too, since he reportedly walked up to 20 miles a day and said he did his best work while strolling around the garden.

Sitting in front of a blank Word document, willing the words to come, is futile. When I'm stuck on how to start a chapter, or how to solve a structuring snafu, or how to pull the right metaphor from deep within my brain, I generally bugger off out into the day or night, and run, swim or simply walk.

The blood flow of exercise pumps up your brain function, Professor Justin Rhodes told the *Scientific American*. 'The hippocampus, a part of the brain critical for learning and memory, is highly active during exercise,' he said. 'When the neurons in this structure rev up, research shows that our cognitive function improves.'

It can even reverse the effects of ageing on the brain, he adds. 'Other recent work indicates that aerobic exercise can actually reverse hippocampal shrinkage, which occurs naturally with age, and consequently boost memory in older adults.'

Nine times out of ten, I come back from my run/walk with the answer, simply from having not directly thought about it for a bit. I'll have been concentrating on placing one foot in front of the other, and not singing out loud to 'One Way or Another' by Blondie, and I'll have to stop, mid-jog, to frantically make a note in my phone; catching the thought by its tail.

Experts call this the 'deliberation-without-attention effect', and the crux of it is that, if you want to solve a complex riddle, give it to your unconscious mind to solve by distracting yourself with something else.

It's become a noughties joke, best exemplified by film *The Internship*, that modern workplaces feature pool tables, slides, scooters and nap-pods. But they're onto something. Because it's often when we're not thinking about work at all, that the best ideas fizz in our brains.

Much as a watched kettle never boils (it does, but let's just suspend disbelief, 'kay?), the watched page, easel, pottery wheel, producing desk, whatever, is something to walk away from.

Whether it's with your body, your hands or your voice, making your brain manifest actual things, no matter how ordinary, is immensely rewarding. And it doesn't matter if anyone else thinks they're good. If they think it's 'nothing to write home about'. Sod them. Why aren't they creating their own things?

ODES TO THE ORDINARY

An ode to artists who pay homage to ordinary things

I chose to open this book with an Andy Warhol quote because he was an icon of the ordinary. A grandmaster at placing the humdrum centre stage. And at making a Campbell's soup can into a great work of art.

I'm as partial to the fantastical as the next person; being fond of Chagall's cello-playing goat (Julia Roberts said it was a violin in *Notting Hill*, but it's a cello sweetie) and macabre circus scenes; or Klimt's flame-haired mermaids with breasts that wouldn't look out of place on a Pirelli calendar; or Botticelli's Venus being birthed by a seashell.

And yet, so much of our most celebrated art is of everyday items, immortalized on canvas. Van Gogh's chair or sunflowers; Hopper's film-noir gas stations and cafes; Hockney's no-nonsense *Fruit on a Bench*.

Meanwhile, Martin Parr is probably the most famous photographer (of many) who are fascinated by workaday folk, exhibiting what *The Times* calls 'an extraordinary eye for the ordinary.' His captures are at once fantastically everyday, yet wonderfully wry.

A teenage boy, whose ice cream lopsides as he stares at the ice-cream vendor's boobs. A camera-bearing tourist with emerald and amethyst pigeons perched on her head. A girl aping a llama. A flock of paradise-bird hatted ladies at the races, all fixated by their phones.

Then there's Mike Leigh's exquisitely quotidian dramas, which thrust NHS counsellors, waitresses, plumbers and working-class mothers onto a plinth, as if a kitchen sink turned modern art.

Most notably for me is his life-affirming work *Happy-Go-Lucky* (a story of a school teacher's indestructible cheerfulness in the face of the bleak, as if *Amelie* were transported to Northern England and stripped of all of its flattering filters).

Tracey Emin also mischievously intersects high art with the banal. Of course, there was *My Bed*, an intimate, confronting portrait of a heartbreak. But less well known is a landscape photo of Tracey sat in a shabby, heirloom armchair juxtaposed against the Mars-like magnificence of Monument Valley; with the motto of her grandma embroidered across it: 'There's a lot of money in chairs'. Indeed, Tracey did make a lot of money from sitting in that particular chair.

Much of our planet's favourite art is actually of homely items; or people who are resplendent in their averageness. An ordinary armchair can be – is – high art.

> 'The true secret of happiness lies in the taking a genuine interest in all the details of daily life, in elevating them by art...'
>
> William Morris

ORDINARY JOYS PART IV

- That it's OK to wave at strangers from the following: boats, open-top buses and tuk-tuks. I don't why this is, but I like it.

- Yellow and orange. (Graphic designer Orlagh O'Brien asked 250 people and found that these colours most strongly evoke joy.)

- Writing your name in the night sky with a sparkler.

- The cheeky white flash of a rabbit's bum, or the swish of a horse's tail.

- Toes in a furry rug.

- Coat hooks that look like a face, or a sozzled octopus.

- The satisfying finality of pulling a handbrake up. Destination, reached.

- The feeling of an animal or child running towards you, with unbridled love.

- Good-natured haggling in a market. Reaching a mutually beneficial price. Shaking on it.

- Watching elderly people nailing a tango, or crushing a waltz. Skills.

- A furry green chestnut dropping from a tree, like an impish miniature alien missile.

- 'Dad joke' gate signs that say things like 'Trespassers will be shot. Survivors will be shot again', or blue plaques announcing 'Nobody famous has ever lived here'.

- An exceptionally well-organized Tupperware drawer, in which no receptacle goes lid-less.

VII: ORDINARY BODIES

IN PRAISE OF AVERAGE ATTRACTIVENESS

I can, at times, look pretty hot. Other times, I'm tepid – 'bung her in the microwave for a minute and we'll see'. Then there are the days when I'm actively minging.

I'm averagely attractive. You probably are too. And that's OK.

We now live in a world where we are much more polished and attractive on our socials catwalk, than we are in real life. We look better in photos than we do in 3D. We slide saturation scales up to make ourselves look more tanned; we whiten teeth by veiling ourselves in a flattering filter; we can even slim our bodies and change our faces, smoothing out wrinkles with a mere click.

Our Instagram stories are our audition tape, our photos are our go-see model portfolio, our status updates are our stand-up comedy, all of which is put out there with the purpose of gaining acceptance, approval and acclaim.

This means that what we actually see in the mirror has become a substandard shadow-twin to the socials self we curate. This is why we can experience a horrified reaction when we accidentally turn our camera to selfie mode.

But the reality is, you're probably better looking than you think, given people tend to underestimate their attractiveness. The authors of *The Beauty Prescription* (Eva Ritvo and Debra Luftman, respectively a psychiatrist and dermatologist) have pinned our underestimation at around 20 per cent.

The imaginary partner comparathon

One thing that fuels a dissatisfaction with the way we look, is the totally fictional belief that our partner is comparing us to a model on telly, or a heavenly body on the street. Errrrm.

I recently realized that I often look at other women as if through a frat-boy male gaze. I imagine that they see women as isolated body parts, as flesh-and-blood wares in a red-light district, when rationally, I know that's highly unlikely. I don't look at men that way. Nor do I ever compare my partner to extraordinary specimens.

Do you? Do you sit there and do a splitscreen of Channing Tatum, or Margot Robbie, with your partner? I bet you don't. So why would they? I also never compare my current partner's body to my exes. Do you? Well, there you go then. It's just a dunderheaded myth, that we're all paranoid about, and yet never do ourselves.

Studies have found that our partner finds us more attractive than strangers do, and that our partner rates us as *more attractive* than we rate ourselves. Comforting. In other surprising attractiveness news, kindness is foxy. Men and women who perform altruistic behaviours appear more attractive to others.

With great beauty, comes great weirdness

A Reddit thread which asked 'conventionally attractive women' for the downsides of being smokin' makes for compulsive reading (and is printed here exactly as it appeared online).

- 'No one takes me seriously. They assume that I'm stupid and even when I prove that I'm not, there's still that feeling. It's even been implied that I'd do best as a trophy wife.'

- 'I have to be careful about going out drinking with male friends. After a few drinks, it's not uncommon for them to get flirty (even if they're in a relationship) and I hate having to find a non-awkward way to shut them down while somehow maintaining our friendship. Is it the most awful thing in the world? No. But I wish it wasn't something I had to constantly worry about.'

- 'I used to get unwanted attention if I dressed up when I was younger, so I "fixed" my walk so that there was no hip swinging, my head was straight, kind of ghost-like gliding, I dressed like a tomboy most of the time, and put no effort in my daily look.'

- 'I'm fairly young (mid-twenties) and have had a hard time advancing in the workplace despite getting more responsibility at work. I was told by the HR person in charge of the hiring committee for the internal transfer I applied for that I didn't have a chance because older male co-workers won't take me seriously and could get distracted. I put in a complaint with the VP of staff and left that job.'

- 'I had multiple professors tell me that they had drastically underestimated me based on my appearance, and pretty much ignored me for the first half of a semester before they began seeing my work.'

- 'Random guys on the street ask me if I want to grab a coffee or give them my number regularly. The negative side effect: creepy old men follow me or try to talk to me in public. They enter my personal space and I am scared.'

Food for thought, no?

Much has been written about the 'beauty premium', whereby hotter people get better societal treatment, but I find the opposite is also true. In that we make unforgiving snap judgements about the genetically gifted.

Think about some extraordinary-looking people that you see around, but you don't know. Do you look at them and think, 'I bet they're really clever and a kind person'. Or do you look at them and think, 'I bet she's a real uppity cow', or 'I bet they're not the brightest crayon in the box', or 'I bet he's obsessed with the gym'.

The dark side of the moon, the flipside of luminous good looks, is that they attract compliments, yes, but they also tend to attract a lot of primordial sexual energy, or unfair presumptions that gorgeousness equals pretentiousness, or snap assumptions that just because he's hench he probably never reads a book.

It's easier to be a six rather than a nine in terms of everyday life. I once saw Scarlett Johansson backstage at Live 8 and she'd done everything she possibly could to look ordinary, to become invisible, by wearing no make-up, a baseball cap and joggers. I didn't even notice her, until someone pointed her out. I doubt she was doing this because she's a celebrity, since the backstage area was heaving with A-listers; Madonna, Sting, The Killers, the Beckhams and Brad Pitt, to name but a few.

Extraordinarily attractive people swaddle their unearthly glow in sunglasses, hats and scarves, not only because they don't want to be recognized if they're famous, but also because they just want to halt the weirdness of random people following them home and asking for their number.

There's also a peculiar link between being top of the attractiveness pile and divorce. One 2017 study found that '...those rated as more attractive in high school yearbooks were married for shorter durations and more likely to divorce'.

The beauty industry is designed to agitate dissatisfaction

I imagine the beauty industry as evil geniuses who sit stroking white cats, going, 'What can we tell them they need, that they *don't have*? Or what do they *have*, that we can tell them is vile and must be eradicated?'

Case in point: the chicanery around eyebrows. Oh the irony (eye-rony?) that women spent the eighties and nineties trying to slim our 'bushy is bad' eyebrows into skinny arches, a la 1990s Gwen Stefani, Drew Barrymore, Kate Moss and Charlize Theron.

Cue early noughties. Enter a dramatic about-face by the cat-stroking beauty industry, and suddenly we are told that eyebrows are the most important feature on our faces.

Now, thin eyebrows are seen as beauty anathema, with *Elle**running skinny-brow-shaming articles such as 'What 26 celebs would look like with '90s brows (spoiler: it's weird)'.

Beauty industry: 'Luckily we have several expensive products for you to buy to solve the problem which we have decided now exists on your face! Behold our range of eyebrow serums, boy-brow pencils, wax, mascara, micro-blading...' *Sweeps hand at products* 'You're welcome!' *Flounces away in a cloud of perfume*

Guess what effect this has? It ker-chings them bucketloads of money as millions of women who dutifully plucked their eyebrows into non-existence, now try to summon them back out of the mists of time, or pretend they are there when they're not.

Men's eyebrows are mostly left well alone, aside from the 'eyebrow' trimmer function on depilation devices that suggests they don't allow them to grow to wizard proportions.

Nonetheless, men don't get off scot-free. Enter the upsurge in grooming products with hilariously macho names, such as 'isotonic power hydration!', 'caffeine dead-lift exfoliator!' (totally just made those up, but the following two are real), 'urban camouflage concealer' and 'lip balm agent'. Anyone would think men are hiding their spots and moisturising their lips while on a secret mission in the jungle. But, this testosterone-pumped marketing works.

They're also marketed nose- and ear-trimmers, for their perfectly healthy nasal/earlug hair that is meant to protect their nose and ears from invasive

---

*I'm absolutely certain *Elle* is one of the very magazines that would have cajoled us into plucking our brows into oblivion way back when.

visitors such as germs, fungus and spores. And on cue, millions of men obediently deny evolution's decision for them to have hair there, by trimming it away, because of an order from the grooming eyries of power.

A pact to drop the 'I'm ugly today' disclaimer

You've done it. I've definitely done it.

Here's how the disclaimer goes: 'I didn't manage to wash my hair, obviously' or 'And I have this horrible spot' or 'I didn't get around to ironing this' and the other person is baffled, because they didn't even notice.

While we are 100 per cent aware of the minutiae of difference in our appearance day-to-day, I would guestimate that other people are only around 20 per cent aware. We see ourselves in a 5× magnified mirror.

The only person who is hyper-aware of what we look like is indeed, ourselves.

AGEING LIKE WE ARE INTENDED TO

I am at that age now where the most common compliment I get is: 'You look great for your age!'

Note 'for your age'. The implication is that my age is bad, and I have done well because I look alright despite it. It's like saying, 'You look lovely – even though you are wearing that dress'. Or: 'You look hot – despite your hairstyle'.

It betrays an entrenched, earth-core-deep belief in our society that ageing is a bad thing, and we need to dodge, defy and sidestep it as best we can.

Why?

The best finding I dug up on our national body image, is that the sexagenarians among us feel the sexiest. Yup, those aged between 60 and 69 are crushing it when it comes to feeling comfortable in their own skin.

Nearly seven in ten reported that they're 'happy with their body' in a 2015 YouGov survey. Doesn't this just go to show that your body image has nothing to do with how bouncy your bottom is, or how taut your tummy, and instead has everything to do with self-acceptance?

The invisibility cloak of age

A common complaint about ageing is starting to feel invisible. If you've once felt very visible to the general public, if you've once attracted stares and compliments and offers of dinner just for walking down the street, it can be unsettling to get older, since it feels like you're gradually being rubbed out by a giant eraser.

My best mate and I recently walked down a street in Barcelona, both wearing our finest, to the grand acclaim of exactly zero attention. 'Do you remember when we used to literally stop traffic?' I said, harking back to the days when men would screech to a halt in the street to entreat us to hand over our contact details.

But, we used to go out practically wearing bikinis, and looking for this attention. Many of those stopped cars were merely looking for one thing from us, and the reason they'd slammed on the brakes to talk to us, was because our bikini-esque clothes were giving them the impression that they might get it.

It's not fair, but it is true. Women should be able to go out topless and be left alone, but they're not, and my friend and I were complicit in this skimpiness/attention exchange. Now we wear clothes that cover us up, because deep down, we want to be left alone, even though we then moan about being left alone.

Great beauty and angst about it are the preserve of the twentysomethings, and I don't miss that one little whit. I used to have a bum like two bowling balls. Now it's more like an overripe peach. And I'm cool with that.

Ten-year challenges

Back when everyone was doing the #10yearchallenge I didn't partake, because it largely seemed to be an exercise in 'Check me out, I defy the ageing process! SAY HOW YOUNG I LOOK'.

None of us defy ageing, nor should we, because ageing is beautiful. Why are we so obsessed with remaining young, in the manner of star-eating harpies from *Stardust*?! We feel tyrannized by the inexorable march of time.

We are supposed to mature, rather than remain cryogenically frozen; our skin is a storyteller, our body gets weighed down with wisdom, our foreheads become lined with the tales of our existence, our smiles leave a concertina of crinkles, our faces soften as our temperaments mellow. Grey hair is actually just translucent. 'Silver hair, don't care' should be 'translucent hair, don't care', but that doesn't have the same ring to it.

When I look at pictures of me now and ten years ago I can see two satisfying things: I look happier and healthier now. I don't look as young now, and I don't give a rat's ass about that, but I do have more of a light in my eyes, because I look after myself and I'm a damn sight happier.

I'm healthier because I self-parent, whereas I used to self-sabotage. I go to bed at 10pm more than 2am. I go for massages rather than to Tiger Tiger. I give my time to people who nourish me, rather than people who are toxic.

Invisibility is a superpower

That invisibility I now feel is freeing. So freeing that when it is punctured, by a stranger making advances, I feel as if my new superpower has rescinded. I find myself metaphorically jiggling the batteries to turn it back on, by spending the next few days in cardigans, leggings and zero make-up.

What if, instead of abhorring this invisibility cloak awarded to us inch-by-inch as we age, we shrugged it on willingly, even with relief? I used to walk down the street and brace whenever I approached a group of beery men given the inevitable comments; now I can dance around them largely without incident, while they gawp at the twentysomething behind me.

I never enjoyed having my tits or ass appraised anyway, as if on *Strictly Come Sexy*, by horny bell-ends. I sought their attention purely because I was desperately insecure. And I'm not anymore. Since the confounding thing is, as our beauty blurs like a once-sharp Indian tapestry softens and frays, our insecurities recede.

Ten years from now I don't want to look ten years younger than I actually am. I want to have even more light in my eyes – and stories, wisdom and smiles written all over my face and body. Bring it on.

Instead of saying I'm 39, I might start saying I'm 'on level 39'. That feels more accurate. Because look how long I've survived, and how I now thrive! Despite repeated attempts to destroy myself.

What level are you on? If you're ahead of me I applaud your game-of-life playing prowess, friend.

> 'It might be a strange irony that the cure for worrying about ageing is sometimes, well, *ageing*.'
>
> Matt Haig, *Notes on a Nervous Planet*

THINGS THAT DIDN'T
HAPPEN IN MY TWENTIES

1. Now, when I drop things on the floor, I do a mental cost/benefit analysis before picking them up.

2. Sometimes when I'm wearing a bra in which my nips are visible, I look down and notice they're looking in different directions. I have to scoop them into seeing straight.

3. When I see an unmade bed, an unwiped surface or an open front door in a film, it bugs me.

4. A deep pool without steps or gradual entry now represents a challenge. Will I be able to get out? Who knows.

5. Thigh gap? More like a thigh crack.

6. When someone comes over, I now spend 50 minutes on my flat and ten on myself, meaning I look like Worzel Gummidge, but my bathroom looks beaut.

7. Elasticated waistbands.

8. Yesterday I got onto a trampoline to show my niece an adventurous move. Turns out my pelvic floor isn't into that one anymore.

9. That mysterious switchover from 'miss' to 'ma'am'.

10. Two words. Back fat. Not a fan.

11. That 'urrg...oof' sound I now appear to need to make in order to get out of the back seat of a car.

HAVING A REGULAR-SIZED BODY

A YouGov survey from a few years back found that 37 per cent of Brits are unhappy with their bodies.

Much of this national body-image crisis can be laid at the door of us comparing ourselves to people online. The same YouGov poll found that 74 per cent say that celebrity culture has a negative impact on women's perception of their bodies. Men's too, I'd bet my bottom dollar.

We are not supposed to be comparing ourselves to the most genetically gold-plated, outrageously talented people on the planet. It's not normal to be fed a tickertape of the earth's most spectacular specimens. As writer John Naish puts it, we're trying to keep up with the 'mythic super-Joneses'.

In hunter-gatherer villages we only compared ourselves to a few dozen – probably at most a hundred – of our local peers. Those within our immediate field of vision; now the race has become global.

'Our social groups used to be much smaller,' says Professor Cregan-Reid, 'and were more real because they were not sanitized by distance and social-media editing.' Our Stone Age brains have not caught up with the fact that social media has now pushed us into a dystopian, cavernous, mega-gym with thousands of others, trying to race the 0.01 per cent of the elite. It's enough to send you totally bonkers. 'But on the upside, we mostly don't have to worry about being eaten by tigers,' adds Professor Cregan-Reid, brightly.

Also, see those beach bikini pictures in the Sidebar of Shame? They have been entirely agreed upon. It's well known in magazine and newspaper circles that celebrities will agree to a set photo shoot with the local paparazzo in order to be left alone the rest of the time.

This answers a lot of modern-day mysteries. Who goes to the beach with long, tousled locks and in full make-up, or stands flexing their guns in the surf? No one, that's who. The rest of the time, these celebs are probably going to the beach just like us: with sweaty slapped-back hair and pink faces encased in a film of SPF 50.

There's a gap between what women think men want, and what they actually want. A 2010 study gathered data from female participants in 26 countries. They asked women to indicate the body shape they thought would be most desirable to men. Across cultures, women thought that men would prefer a thinner body size than the men *actually preferred*.

And surgery to narrow the gap between them and us doesn't generally scratch the unhappy itch. A review of seven separate studies found that women who have had breast enlargements are two to three times more likely to commit suicide, when compared to those who had no surgery.

Many women think having Double-Ds will cure our bodily neuroses, but they do no such thing. Because – hedonic adaptation. We find something else we want to change, once we hop aboard that dangerous nip-tuck escalator.

Making peace with my ordinary body

In general, I have been fortunate in the size department. I've inherited my father's daddy-long-legs frame, and ability to seemingly eat my way through my twenties and thirties as if Desperate Dana at a pie-eating contest, with little more than slight fluctuations.

However, my metabolism is clearly tired of all of that furnacing, because I was a size 8 in my teens, a 10 in my twenties and thirties, and I am undoubtedly now a 12.

I arrived at this conclusion because I found myself always having to undo jeans and skirts while sitting down. This is not normal. This is the kind of palaver that leads to you standing up in Pizza Express and finding that your little silk skater skirt (with pockets, love it when they have pockets) is now a puddle around your ankles.

I have now finally wised up, given my least-forgiving size 10s to charity, and bought some magnanimous size 12s instead. Because life's too short to wear clothes that stop you from eating three courses comfortably, squeeze your spleen and that you have to remember to re-button.

I know that being a size 12 is no big deal, it is indeed, a total non-deal. However, what I'm saying is this: I have now just totally accepted that my body wanted to be 9.5 stone at 18, 10 stone at 25, 10.5 stone at 30 and knocking on 11 stone now.

I am now exactly the average weight of your regular British woman, at 11 stone. And yet, we're all sold this idea that anything over 10 stone (or a size 10) is a failure. It's propaganda, and we should wholeheartedly reject it.

Men, meanwhile, may be surprised to learn that the average British male is 13 stone, doesn't have #shredded abs you can store small stationery items in, and is 5ft 9in, not 6 foot, as is commonly believed.

You know best, body. Do your thing. I'll just carry on eating healthily (sortof, aside from ~~sinful~~ divine lemon cheesecake in glass ramekins; my local glass-recycling bin knows of my Gü habit) and exercising, and you crack on being whatever size you wanna be.

Your body knows what to do, so let it. And, irrespective of what those gym-militants say about your weight being entirely within your control ('Eat less, move more' they parrot, while I nod sweetly and have dark fantasies about pushing them into the pool), the experts say different.

Timothy Frayling, a professor of human genetics at the University of Exeter (who probably knows better than your mate), has been quoted as saying that our BMI is influenced by genetics up to 70 per cent. This is based on studies of twins raised separately.

Yes, what we do makes some difference, but it can't make the dramatic difference promised by chirpy celebs bouncing around on fitness DVDs. Biological determinism is real.

Let's all stop trying to be a size 10 (or less). And yes, size 10 is indeed extraordinary, given the average British woman is a beautiful size 16.

In search of perfect genitalia

There is now a disturbing array of ways you can upgrade your genitals. Vajazzles were one thing; now there are vajacials. Vaginal steaming anyone?

You can even have your anus bleached. 'I love my new anus!' cries Helen in *Bridesmaids*. I'm still not entirely sure what a bleached anus is, and I'm too scared to Google it.

We live in a society where women regard hairless, airbrushed vaginas from porn and have surgery to mimic them; risking losing their ability *to orgasm* in order to reduce the size of their perfectly lovely labia. I read one dreadful story in which a woman went to have her labia reduced and ended up with *no labia*. Yeesh.

We live in a society where 'Big Dick Energy' is used as shorthand for swagger by writers in papers who think of themselves as right-on, and yet, imagine what message that gives vulnerable adolescent boys. 'Big Tit Energy' would trigger an outcry, and yet BDE is allowed to exist, and even thrive.

It's unbelievably wonky. We need to protect our boys as much as we do our girls, from messaging like this; that their body parts need to be a certain size.

Listen up, guys. It's commonly cited that most of the vagina's nerve endings are in the first couple of inches. Which means women are generally truly, madly, deeply cool with whatever size you bring.

Plus, the largest-ever study of its type found that only 18 per cent of women orgasm through penetration alone. Women need clitoral stimulation for their orgasms, much more than intercourse. What you *do* is actually a lot more important than size.

Forgiving your feet

Female shoe shops predominately display dainty size 5s, which if we're the national average of 6.5 (in the sixties, it was size 4), gives us the impression that our feet are abnormally large.

I'm a size 7, barely a whisker above the average and yet, I always feel like an *insert circus music* clown-footed giant, given I have to ask for my size, as if I am an unusual shoe-wearer. I imagine them going out to a special hangar in the back, where they have to keep the size 7s and up.

Meanwhile men are told they need to have big feet, because big feet means a…which brings us back to the absolute fiction that women have to be impaled in order to receive pleasure. Nope.

Run-of-the-mill gnashers

A 2018 survey found that four in ten Brits are unhappy with the way their teeth look. Every now and then somebody will compliment me on my teeth, and I will have to stop myself from saying, 'Are you demented?!' and swiping at their compliment in the manner of a toddler sending a spear of asparagus airborne. 'Thank you,' I say, utterly unconvinced and checking for hidden cameras.

Having conducted a totally unscientific study by asking all of my friends, including those with the very nicest teeth in my eyes, I have concluded that all of us have dental dysmorphia.

'What about this bit here, where they overlap,' said Leila, or 'I just want Hollywood star veneers,' said Josh, or 'They're just too big,' said Katie.

When people point out a fatal tooth flaw they want to have fixed, how often have we actually noticed it? Rarely. My theory is that we only ever notice if people have particularly grim or particularly dazzling teeth. Middlin' teeth just slide by unnoticed. Aside from in our own heads.

ODES TO THE ORDINARY
An ode to midlife

'Middle age' has been replaced with 'Midlife', which I thunderously applaud. 'Middle-aged', for me, always evoked the 'Middle Ages' (otherwise known as the 'Dark Ages'), summoning forth dusty relics and the fall of an empire.
No, ta.

When I was 19, I remember thinking that people who were approaching 40 were practically dead. I also recall thinking that people in their late thirties no doubt acutely envied my youth, and surely longed to switch places with me via some magical filmic device; perhaps an enchanted fountain at midnight, Zoltar the bearded fortune-telling dude, or a spell from a pissed-off gypsy, like in all those age-switching Hollywood films (of which *Big* is the pinnacle, obviously).

However, I have absolutely zero desire to go back to 19, or 29 or even 35. What about you? If you were given a portal into a younger body and life, right now? Straight back to that career ledge, bank account and mental health?

Often we think the answer would be 'hell yeah', but when it comes to the crunch *beckons you towards the portal I just ripped out of thin air* you wouldn't actually accept the invitation. 'And go through all that again? Errr...'

The myth that our high school days are the best of our lives, when they're usually torture c/o hormones, is only topped by the other youth-worshipping claim; that our twenties are a blast. I mean, they are sometimes, but they're also colossally frustrating and petrifying too.

It's usually upwards of 30 when true contentment really beds in. A recent study by the University of Alberta found that people tend to be happier when they're 40, than they were when they were 18.

'Psychologists call this the paradox of ageing,' says Professor Cregan-Reid. 'As the body fails, the general psychological outlook of the individual improves.'

As Phoebe Waller-Bridge said on Elizabeth Day's *How to Fail* podcast, 'I'd really like to have the skin from my twenties, but I prefer my heart and my guts now'. Our twenties are a dewy-skinned baptism of fire, in which we're forged. We have to be bouncy-limbed to survive them.

'Midlife' also more explicitly acknowledges that *we're only halfway through people*. A very handy life expectancy calculator from the Office of National Statistics (see Sources on page 257 for the URL) has just told me that I'm expected to live until 89. The calculator comfortingly adds, 'That's 50 years from now'. Thanks calculator! Zoiks. Fifty whole years.

Let's stick a pin in the socially hawked notion that you need to do/achieve everything by 50, since after that you're basically plodding towards the exit sign. At 50, you're a youngster in the grand scheme of things.

There is so much time left. Time to travel, paint, get a cockatoo and teach it French, learn to juggle; whatever it is you want to do. *So much time.*

'At age 20, we worry about what others think of us. At age 40, we don't care what they think of us. At age 60, we discover they haven't been thinking of us at all.'

Ann Landers, advice columnist

EXERCISING FOR YOUR BRAIN, RATHER THAN YOUR BUM

'It ain't about the ass, it's about the brain.'

Lena Dunham

Coming back to my graduation from size 10 to size 12, the way it also shifted my attitude to exercise turned up a surprising revelation. Up until then, I'd never exercised in order to lose weight. I enjoyed exercising. It wasn't a chore. I didn't struggle to motivate myself.

I suddenly started exercising for a different reason, and found that working out became an entirely different animal. Most notably, I was exercising *less*. I had to drag myself out for runs, rather than bouncing out for them.

Mystifying. And frustrating.

For answers, I turned to the work of the brilliant Dr Michelle Segar, a motivation scientist from the University of Michigan, and the author of *No Sweat: how the simple science of motivation can bring you a lifetime of fitness*.

Dr Segar and her colleagues undertook a study to find out how our motivations for exercise affect our engagement in it. From their pool of participants, 75 per cent were exercising for weight loss (or better health), while 25 per cent exercised to enhance well-being or feel more centred.

They then followed the exercise patterns of both groups over the next year. And guess what? The first group – those who were lacing up their trainers in order to lose weight – spent the *least amount of time* exercising. Those who exercised for their mental health alone – rather than a smaller ass – exercised 32 per cent more.

This is echoed in many other studies. In more research that Dr Segar cites, exercisers were defined as 'body-shapers' or 'non body-shapers'. The 'non body-shapers' exercised 40 per cent more.

Basically, exercising for weight loss slays your buzz. 'If you find that exercise feels like a chore, then it's because you feel like you *should*, rather than you *want to*,' says Dr Segar. Personally, I think the *should* motivation also wakes up our surly teenage anarchists, who want to give *what we should do* the finger and go and smoke weed instead.

It all makes sense. Because as soon as I stopped caring about the graduation to size 12, I started enjoying exercise again.

I started noticing once more how running has the ability to take my mood from a four to an eight, rather than thinking, 'I've only run 5km, need to run more to lose tapas I ate last night!'

Running is for me, mental alchemy. Pre-run I will be slouching about, thinking, 'Life not fair. Hate life.' Mid-run, I am bowling down a country lane, air-drumming like a deranged monkey to Metallica's 'Enter Sandman'. Post-run, I feel like liquid gold is running through my veins.

When my size became irrelevant once more, I remembered how I sleep like a sparked-out toddler after a swim, rather than bullying myself into doing a kilometre in the pool. And I recalled that yoga is like a mini-break for my manic mind, rather than 'work' for my core.

And hey presto; I started exercising five times a week again.

The reason exercise has the ability to lift our mood so dramatically, is because it is a smash-grab at the pharmacy of feelgood chemicals that already exist in our brain. Drugs and pills work because they tap into things that are already there. We can provoke them naturally through exercise, says neuroscientist Dr Korb. 'Endorphins are the brain's own form of morphine,' he says, 'while endocannabinoids are the brain's own form of cannabis.'

We don't need a dealer or a prescription to get *high*. All we need is to move our bodies, with the motive of feeling good, rather than looking good.

ODES TO THE ORDINARY

An ode to showers

I used to think of self-care as a necessary evil. Now I undertake these bodily chores with a regard for my body I just didn't have before. Because I know of the power they can have on our mental health.

It's like Hannah Jane Parkinson wrote in the *Guardian* about coming out of a psychiatric ward and discovering a 'wholesome resetting' joy in the quotidian act of spending 15 minutes brushing her teeth, a ritual replete with a tongue brush and a dye that highlights plaque.

Producing the effect where, when she runs her tongue across her teeth, 'they feel as though they are made of silk,' writes Parkinson. 'These tiny grooming actions we perform can somehow make a big difference when we feel like crap'.

And that's what it's about – the self respect to say you're worth a £1 face mask from Boots. Or grating your hard feet and slathering on silky foot cream. Or for men, treating yourself to an old-fashioned barber's shave.

As with cleaning, sometimes outside differences cause internal subsidence to settle. When the floor we are standing on is mopped and the feet are less gnarly, it can make us feel more grounded and secure.

YOU ARE *SUPPOSED* TO HAVE HAIR THERE

It's utterly ordinary to have bodily hair in places we are told we are not supposed to.

Razor adverts aimed at women traditionally never ever feature actual leg hair, or armpit hair, or bikini line hair, because it would be regarded as visually offensive. We now have sanitary protection adverts that feature red, rather than blue, 'blood', but we still don't have women actually shaving. Think of how strange that is, when you compare it to male razor adverts. Imagine a male shaving advert that featured zero actual stubble.

For women, the word that most often precedes stubble is 'unsightly'. Not only are we expected to remove the hair that naturally occurs over a third of our body, we are also expected to remove it so effectively that it looks like we never grow hair there.

Men can legitimately leave stubble, because duh, they have hair there. Men can display regrowth, whereas ours is regarded as anathema to femininity.

Guys, imagine this for a moment. Imagine you want to go for a swim and, in order to go for a socially endorsed one, you need to take a razor to a third of your body. At least. Truly try to imagine that.

'But it's not as if I could grow a big messy beard like Dumbledore, I need to keep my facial hair trim,' protested one male friend when I pointed this out. Er, yes you could? Have you *been* to East London recently, buddy?! A wizardy beard is practically a status symbol.

Besides, the two are far from the same. Facial hair is a twentieth of the surface area of the body hair women are expected to remove.

Billie, an American brand, lobbed the rulebook out of the window last year by becoming the first razor brand in the world to put out an advert that didn't feature exclusively hairless women. Their brilliant ad opened on a fluffy pink mule and panned up to a full leg of hair, showing a woman with multi-coloured nails lovingly caressing a navel trail, another casually hairdrying her pit hair, a badass monobrow, and a woman shaving just the ripped sections of her jeans (yup). Those who made this advert are straight-up legends.

We are not hairless geishas

I remember being utterly dismayed as a teen that even after I shaved with the best razor available in the late nineties (with three blades!) and the pink shaving foam which bloomed on my wet hand like a rainforest flower on time-lapse film, that it was still obvious that *I had hair there*. I still had a smattering of pepper on my ankles, as if I was a seasoned turkey.

This wouldn't do, as I *wasn't supposed to have hair there*. So I started shaving my legs so savagely that I would have little red dots instead (but at least there was no evidence of hair) and plastering foundation all over my legs.

My hair removal was undertaken entirely to win the approval of the male gaze, but it was also policed by other women. 'You may want to take a look at that,' a female friend would say, gesturing to my bikini line.

In the nineties, female depilation was still regarded as a shame-faced thing to be undertaken entirely in private. I had one boyfriend who yelped, horrified, 'Ugh, don't tell ME that,' when I mentioned that I needed to shave my legs before we went to bed. Further compounding my belief that my leg hair was an abomination which should be removed without his knowledge, for fear it may decimate his desire for me.

In 2011, Caitlin Moran published *How to Be a Woman*, in which she described running her fingers through her pubic hair. 'Lying on a hammock, gently finger-combing your Wookie whilst staring up at the sky is one of the great pleasures of adulthood,' she wrote. Moran went on to describe a full bush as something grown women ought to be proud of, rather than ashamed.

'A lovely furry moof that looks – when she sits, naked – as if she has a marmoset sitting in her lap. A tame marmoset, that she can send off to pickpocket things, should she so need it – like that trained monkey in *Raiders of the Lost Ark*.'

I was 31, and it was the first time I had heard a woman talk about her bikini wildgrowth as glorious, rather than gruesome. It felt radical then, this idea that maybe we don't have to be hairless geishas who bow and defer, and to a certain extent it still does now, as the norm is still for women to pretend that they have no hair, other than on their heads.

I remember strolling around a canalside market wearing a summer dress and eating an ice cream, when my boyfriend of the time stopped and crooked his finger to beckon my face closer to his. I obliged, thinking he was going to cup my face and say something romantic.

Instead, he pinched a centimetre-long white whisker, yanking it from my cheek and said, 'I like you a lot, but I like you better without that in your face'. He did it in a matter-of-fact way, and I laughed without shame, but the 'I like you better without' stayed with me. 'Without'. Gotcha. I bought a weapons-grade magnifying mirror and the best steel tweezers money can buy, and started a daily patrol on my visage.

Teaching our little boys that girls have hair

I recently had an exchange with a twelve-year-old boy that went like this:

Him: 'I have hairs in my armpits.'
Me: 'Cool! So do I.'
Him: 'Girls don't have hairs in their armpits.'
Me: 'Yes they do, they just often shave it off.'
Him: 'Ugh.'
Me: 'Not ugh, it's natural. You have body hair there and so does everyone else, whatever gender.'
Him: 'Ok. Can I see?'
Me: 'I've shaved it off but you can still see the little bumps.'
Him: 'Huh.'

I realized that the razor-bumps moment meant that I was simultaneously teaching him something important, hopefully smashing a perception for him, that *girls don't have hair there*, but also, given all I had to show him were tiny razor bumps, like mole mounds being evidence of absent moles, I was also teaching him I was ashamed of having hair in my armpits.

I see influencers like artist Florence Given posting gorgeous pictures of themselves in a leopard-print bikini with a downy dusting of armpit hair, and no mention of it in the caption, because now it's officially no big deal, and her followers tell her she's like a 'fucking human highlighter'.

That would not have happened 20 years ago. Remember when Julia Roberts hit the red carpet sporting hairy armpits back in the nineties – headlines! *So many headlines.*

My favourite story about my friend Kate is this one. One day, her husband exclaimed, 'Jesus, what on earth are you doing?!' when he saw her shaving her toes, after a dozen-plus years of him not knowing about her toe-shaving. And she turned to him, deadpan, and said, 'Look at your feet'. He did. 'You have hairs on your feet, and so do I. Because I am human, like you.'

Men are beginning to be dragged into this depilation dictatorship too, with the advent of totally waxed men on TV. I sincerely hope the identikit *Love Island* clone-producing factory doesn't stick around for long enough to influence my ten-year-old nephew. Because women truly do not expect – or even necessarily want – that tanned, ripped hairlessness.

We need to stop hiding that *we have hair there*. Adults all have pubes because, as the name suggests, we have undergone puberty. It is personal choice whether to remove it, but let's stop letting little boys grow up under the misguided notion that women are naturally hairless.

I've now embraced my perfectly natural body hair as utterly normal. I do choose to remove the vast majority of my hair still, so I'm not putting my body where my beliefs are. But I do now go to play tennis with peppery ankles because, d'yknow what, I'm going to play tennis, not appear in a pageant.

Some women have very fair bodily hair; silky gossamer that swoons at the very sight of a razor. I only know one natural blonde like that. One. In fact, she's the only natural blonde I know too. *She* is extraordinary. The rest of us are just beautifully ordinary.

Meanwhile, the reason 'back waxes' are on the depilation menu of every beauty salon from here to Timbuktu is because it's unbelievably ordinary for men to have a dusting on their shoulders. If it wasn't, why would they offer that service?

Here's the reality, for whatever gender. If you keep it clean and trim, everyone will be happy. If they want it Barbie doll/Ken doll bare, they should probably go and audition for *Love Island* and leave you alone.

And if someone asks you to remove all of your body hair before they will consider having sex with you, politely and archly request the same of them.

ODES TO THE ORDINARY
An ode to massages

I have wandered wide-eyed into the consumerist la-la land of seeking the extraordinary spa treatment. I have been caressed with crystals and beaten with bamboo sticks. I have been micro-needled and wrapped in seaweed.

Here's what I've learnt, in my privileged tour through spa treatments (as a result of being a magazine writer who got sent to try this gubbins for free).

Nothing beats a standard massage, and before you shout at me that massages are extraordinary experiences, you can get them on Groupon for as little as £20. You'd spend £20 on a night down the pub, no?

Massages are the only spa treatment that truly gives bang for the buck. And yet, I still keep forgetting this and being led down the garden path into a 'flower bath' where I lie with tiny drowning insects, bemused as to why this is meant to be fun, or a 'The Works' manicure, where my nails essentially look the same, they're just a different colour is all.

I've seen utterly convincing research on massages published in the *International Journal of Neuroscience* (yes, I am that geeky) showing that massages have the power to decrease your cortisol (the stress hormone) by 31 per cent. And to pull serotonin (the happy chemical) up by the bootstraps by 28 per cent. I haven't seen any such research on body scrubs or clay wraps, as glamorous as they sound.

Marketing is a clever sleight of hand, and we fall for it all the time. Personally, I'm going to be sticking to the ordinary, but effective, massages.

IN DEFENCE OF THE BOG-STANDARD WORK OUT

In an effort to get fit like an A-lister, I have boinged around on mini trampolines, plié-ed with all the grace of a gorilla along ballet bars, squatted on vibrating plates, punched the air while spinning to a live saxophonist and poured salt water through my nasal cavity at a yoga retreat.

Things I am yet to try include: being suspended in what amounts to a stork's hammock, yoga with a confetti cannon and press-ups on a floating platform in a London lake.

And of course, there are Pelotons. Which are just really, really fancy exercise bikes. Comedian Clue Heywood rinsed the ridiculousness of Peloton bike adverts in the most perfect way. Here are some of his tweets:

🐦 I put my Peloton bike in the center of the panoramic living room window in my New York penthouse.

🐦 Probably the worst thing about putting a Peloton bike in my spotless huge kitchen is when my dumb kid interrupts the workout. Where is Consuela? She has one job!

🐦 My bright and airy sunroom is a great place for the Peloton bike. I leave the arcadia door ajar so I feel like I'm actually riding a bicycle...outside!

🐦 My Peloton is in the living room because it's my favourite work of art aside from the turquoise marble peacock I keep in the fireplace.

So far, so absurd.

We dream of home gyms decked out with things like Pelotons, and yet the millions of Britons who do invest, mostly use the equipment to hang 'not dirty, but not clean' clothes on, like an outrageously expensive clothes horse. And a fifth of Brits who own an exercise bike, admit to only having used it once.

I'm all for an unusual work out, and yet, I always come back to my very ordinary pursuits of running, yoga, cycling on an actual bike and swimming lengths in a no-frills public leisure centre, complete with soggy plasters and squawking kids (who probably don't buy the story about their wee turning the water pink). Why? Because ordinary is just as good, if not better, and certainly a lot bloody cheaper.

Do exercise you like

It's really important to like the exercise you choose, rather than just doing it because it's a fad, because it gave Daniel Craig his Bond body, or because your mate is. 'Leading neuroscientist Kent Berridge found that "liking" a specific behaviour triggers "wanting" to perform that action,' says motivation scientist Dr Segar.

Far from expensive trainers being desirable, research carried out by biomechanics expert Hannah Rice at the University of Exeter found that pricey, cushioned trainers increased the likelihood of injury. Which brings new meaning to the phrase 'All the gear and no idea'.

We'd actually be better off running barefoot, some sources tell us, but barefoot living is seen as the oddball choice of hippies wearing shirts knitted from beansprouts, or tipsy teenagers who can't walk in their five-inch diamante heels come 1am.

We pay £15 to slog between hammering a treadmill and grunting our way through 20 push-ups (T-Rex style, with our underworked arms), while some hench MC yells at us to go 'faster, harder, more', when one of the very best low-impact ways of staying fit is simply – walking.

Walking is underrated, says Dr Segar. 'Research shows we burn about the same calories training by walking, as we do on a cross-trainer, if we do it at the same intensity and length of time.'

'The easiest kind of movement is that which our ancestors would have done. Physical activity as part of their working day,' says evolution specialist, Professor Cregan-Reid. Walking to and from work, standing desks, that kinda thing. 'They didn't come home at 7pm and then grab a gym bag and go to lift weights, so that's why it's so hard for us to do so too.'

It is hard. Dr Segar explains why: as the shadows grow longer, our willpower gets shorter. 'Studies show that willpower is like sand running through an hour glass,' she says. 'We have a finite amount of self-control, so the more we use it, the less we have.' This means that once you get home from work, your willpower is flashing red, and your self-control is running on empty.

This is accelerated if you emphasize the 'work' in work out, she says. 'Framing a behaviour as work (an obligation) makes the experience of the behaviour more depleting, when compared with those who saw the behaviour as fun,' Dr Segar explains.

What's more, those who drag themselves around out of a sense of obligation, are more likely to scarf junk food afterward. In one study that Dr Segar cites, half of the women in a group were sent on a walk 'for exercise', while the other half were told their walk was 'for fun'. They were then all given unlimited access to M&Ms (sounds like a nice dream I once had). The 'for exercise' group ate twice as many M&Ms as the 'for fun' group.

High intensity produces less pleasure

HIIT? Ugh. I too have been swept along with the obsession with high intensity interval training.

I have done burpees until I would gladly throw myself under a bus rather than do another burpee; I have said 'I can't because I'm nearly 40, and the rest of this class is about 23' to a personal trainer asking me to jump repeatedly onto a thigh-high box; and I have then spent the next two days in excruciating pain, practically doubled over like a fairytale witch who lives in the woods, which apparently is called 'DOMS' (Delayed Onset Muscle Soreness).

I stopped HIITing, because it hurt. It sucked all of the fun out of exercising. And that's not my imagination. Leading exercise psychologist Panteleimon Ekkekakis (is it just me or does he sound like a Philip Pullman character?) has produced a fascinating body of research that shows high intensity exercise tends to *decrease* pleasant feelings. 'The harder someone exercises, in general, the more their pleasure decreases,' confirms Dr Segar.

But she wonders if there might be differences between genders on this question, with men benefitting from high intensity exercise more than women. 'In one study of over 6,000 adults, high-intensity activity was linked to lower depression and anxiety among men, whereas with women, their emotional well-being was boosted with lower-intensity movement,' says Dr Segar.

It also might be that those who choose to go hell-for-leather independently – rather than feeling forced into it by the pace of the class – enjoy it more. Like those ~~maniacs~~ heroes who do the six-day, 125km Marathon des Sables. 'When people decide on their own to exercise at high intensities, they experience less displeasure than when it is imposed upon them,' says Dr Segar.

The upshot of it all is this. Do exercise you like. Do it early in the day. Expensive kit is not necessary. Walking totally counts. And don't go at it too hard, unless you're a person who genuinely loves doing so. OK? OK. I'm off for a nice stroll in my cheap trainers.

A LETTER TO MY BODY

Dear body,

I'm sending you a promise.

I am not going to shoehorn you into too-small trousers anymore, in the act of chasing the extraordinary smugness of being a size 10. So, you can exhale.

I will no longer burn you in the pursuit of a tan I have been marketed into wanting, while far away in the East women bleach their skin doing the exact opposite.

I won't ever squeeze you into too-small shoes again.

I won't make you bleed, in my quest to pretend *I don't have hair there.*

And I promise never to put you under a cosmetic knife, because you are perfectly imperfect just the way you are.

Catherine

THE UNDER-APPRECIATED JOYS OF ORDINARY EXERCISE

1. In mile two you will feel like death could be imminent. But in mile three you will be rewarded by superhero-magnitude endorphins.

2. That moment when you realize that nobody is looking at your Shar Pei puppy stomach in shoulder stand. They're too busy looking at their own.

3. Free-wheeling on a bike past a stationary snarl of a traffic jam. Buh-bye.

4. In the gym, finding that *that* weight no longer challenges you, and the trill of triumph you feel from oh-so-casually reaching for the next couple of kilos up.

5. In spinning, after the acute fear that *you will never be able to clip into the bike*, that kindred, primal togetherness you feel with absolute strangers.

6. The lying-down bit after yoga, or Pilates, or anything mat based. Unbeatable. Leave me here. I'll live here, happily.

7. There is *no better hair-wash* than the one when your hair is thick with sea salt, or clogged with chlorine. Doing it twice, just because.

8. The go-faster surge you get from the opening bars of a song you love. Shout-singing along in empty fields in the countryside.

9. The supremely clean feeling you get from leaving the gym and walking past the two-metre perimeter of ale'n'ash that surrounds the nearby pub. Nope. Not tonight.

VIII: AN ORDINARY
KINDA CONCLUSION

TWEETS FROM PLANET EXTRAORDINARY

If you're still in any doubt that living an extraordinary life inoculates you from feeling short-changed, check out these absolutely real tweets from the insanely privileged.*

(Some of which were likely tongue-in-cheek, but some of which definitely weren't.)

🐦 Nyehhh! I hate having to dress myself!

🐦 Need coffee bad. Wish my Labradoodle could make coffee.

🐦 It's really hard to take selfies in the car when your windows aren't tinted.

🐦 Wearing dry clean only clothes. Driver late. Rain.

🐦 Busy day at fashion. Too tired to paint toenails. Now have to get up at 9am to do them. Honestly.

🐦 No fennel left at the deli. Disaster.

🐦 The maid tidied all my clothes and now I can't find my goddamm Vuitton scarf.

🐦 You brought me into this universe so the LEAST YOU CAN DO is buy me a f*cking iPhoneXS.

🐦 No fresh green juice at Whole Foods. Get your act together LA. I didn't move here so I could drink FRUIT smoothies.

🐦 Don't talk to me during my massage. Just don't.

🐦 Just been asked if I'm a model for twentieth time today by a pathetic man I would never date. YES. Now go. Away.

🐦 Why can't I rent swans for my wedding? Why?

🐦 This Cristal is NOT chilled and all The Help has vanished. JESUS.

🐦 Well, it's official. Our jet-ski is broken.

---

* Twitter handles are obscured to protect the spoilt rotten.

MY MANIFESTO FOR NEVER LOSING ORDINARY JOY

'Ordinary joy' is more than just a way to be happier, for me. My life literally depends on my ability to hang onto it.

It's true that suicide hasn't even flitted across my mind, like a micro-frown across a benign face (blink and you'll miss it), since 2013. But what's also true, is that if we did/thought something before, we can do/think it again.

My continued happiness is an activity I need to engage in, and involves a set of tools I need to pick up and use regularly, like kitchen implements. I have become the kind of person that interjects a conversation with, 'Oh my, what a beautiful cow!', but only because I have now *trained my brain* to seek out glossy chocolatey cows that look like moving Swiss chocolate adverts.

My pessimistic 'What's the point! We're all going to hell in a handcart!' brain has only become a self-made optimist, because of all the work, the adjusting, the writing of gratitudes, and the coaching of it off the sofa and back into the sun. My brain is like a fitness 'before' and 'after' picture. There was a fuckload of work in between those two, to make it happen, that people just don't see.

So, here it is. Exactly what I do now, to hang onto my ordinary joy, to keep myself upright, to stop myself from folding over, and concertina-ing down into deflated negativity once more.

I like to call it the GrayCat method.*And some of it may work for you too, if you relate.

'Better' is an ever-moving target

I recently sat and watched a couple complain bitterly, while I was on (an admittedly extraordinary) holiday. They were a table back from being beachfront in the restaurant, and they were *not flamin' having it*.

All of the tables that looked directly onto the beach were already occupied with other people, who had gotten there first. So, to move this vexed couple, would have meant moving other people. I watched them whinge about their lot with utter recognition and empathy, as I have *been there*.

---

* Like the KonMari method? No? Don't worry, I am indeed totally taking the piss out of myself.

They were a mere six feet further away from the beach, and given they were so intent on fixing that flaw, they were totally forgetting to feel happiness about being in beach utopia.

Thing is, there's always a better table, a better villa, a better sunlounger, a better partner, a better job, a better house, a better everything. And hankering after what we don't have, rather than cherishing what we do, is an unhappy place to live. Hankering is a town you should shoot straight through, rather than stop and unpack at.

Given I am a 'maximizer' by DNA (see page 23 for a reminder), I have to give myself geo- and time-constraints to stop myself from 'bettering' myself into a straitjacket. 'Only look for second-hand bikes for sale within two miles, Cath' for instance, rather than browsing through 29 pages of bikes on Ebay. Or 'Only spend five hours on this piece of work', to avoid finding myself still there, still working, maximizing myself into an early grave at 3am.

On the other hand, if you're a 'satisficer' by nature (see page 23), I applaud you. Because it's seen as uncool to be delighted with the humdrum in life, because we live in a society that says 'no, not that shelf, reach for the higher one!' it's one of the most radical things you can do, *not reaching*, if you don't want to.

The toil/pleasure principle

There is no such thing as easy street, and even if there were, we wouldn't want to live there. Because pleasure is only delicious when it comes after toil. It ceases to feel as exquisite without the struggle as its counterpoint. Ease is only luxurious when framed by something difficult.

Remember the lottery winners and how they lost their ability to enjoy 'mundane pleasures'? Remember how Kanye is most likely just as pissed off as you?

We think we want certain things, but if we had them, they would soon lose their shine. We only get that Friday feeling because of the working week. We only enjoy getting home because we don't spend all of our time in it. We only sigh with pleasure when we curl up with a hot water bottle because we froze our tits off on the walk home.

Buying new clothes is a luxury, because we have a limited budget to do so. Eating French fries with mayo is a naughty joy because we limit our snarfing of them. The first shower after a festival is nirvana via showerhead, because we got really grubby. And the best toilet break is after a savagely long drive on the motorway.

The toil/pleasure principle means that traditionally 'bad' states like being cold, dirty, or busting for a wee, transmute into unabashed pleasure. Once you take away those limits, that contrast, these everyday pleasures cease to have meaning and pleasure.

I once knew a trust-fund kid who got a takeaway practically every night and therefore the 'treat' of having a takeaway was completely lost on her. It was just her dinner. Her 'pleasure' set slider is located higher than the rest of us, because of her privileged circumstances.

Without the toil/pleasure polarity, you're left with the 'so what?' entitlement of a child star, of an aimless existence overstuffed with leisure time and shopping money, and not enough denial and restraint to polarize it against.

Adversity makes us happier, overall

Imagine you have just been born. And have been presented with a clipboard allocating you with two life choices (newborn-you can also read, in this hypothetical, okay?). The two paths are 'Nothing bad ever happens', or 'Shit happens'. We would all, wouldn't we, choose the former box?! With nothing bad ahead. It's a no-brainer.

And yet, adversity is the fire that forges us and more importantly, gives us the capacity to spark joy when good shit does happen. Professor of Psychology Sonja Lyubomirsky says that research shows people who have experienced *some* adversity are happier than those who have experienced no adversity at all. We need the bitter to taste the sweet. The grind to release the relief.

'Contrast is important,' Professor Lyubomirsky agrees. 'It brings in that philosophical notion that we can't know happiness until we've experienced unhappiness. Kids who are exposed to no allergens are more likely to develop allergies to things like peanuts. Our body needs a little stress to build up our psychological immune system.'

If you've experienced childhood trauma, the slap around the face of grief, the ground-vanishing of a break-up, the sudden loss of a home, or the hypnotic and deathly sway of addiction, you'll doubtless have heard the glib cliché 'What doesn't kill you makes you stronger'. But, it really does. You're a survivor. You got through that, so imagine what you can do *now*, with that true grit at your disposal.

If I'm depressed, I move. Pronto.

Back in my darkest times, when I was trying to quit drinking and failing repeatedly, I was once sitting in my parents' garden on a gloriously sunny day, secretly drinking, secretly hating myself, secretly contemplating how to engineer a life exit. I texted a recovery friend and she replied: 'Get up. Move. Do anything. Sort the sock drawer. Mop a floor. Go for a walk. It doesn't matter what you do, just *do something*'.

She was right. When our body is moving, our minds are so much less likely to roam into the netherworld of nihilism.

It's like that amazing scene from *Lost** (sorry non-*Lost* fans, but I will explain) where we watch an unidentified man jumping out of bed, entering a code into a bleeping computer, and then embarking upon a killer morning routine. He puts on some vinyl – loud – cleans some dishes, does some cycling and chin-ups, showers, makes a smoothie and then gets dressed. #Morninggoals

And then we discover that this bloke (Desmond) is stuck in an underground bunker, and his only purpose in life is to push a few buttons every 108 minutes.

'Why did he bother doing all of that?!' I squeaked when I watched it, as a twentysomething with the emotional maturity of a teen. 'All he had to do was lie down and press some buttons!' That was my idea of a dream job. Silly man, doing all that *stuff*.

The difference between me and Desmond, was that Desmond had figured out that productivity and effort are what actually makes us happy. He'd figured out that action and routine are where it's at, so even if he was going to die in a bunker re-setting some weird-ass clock to supposedly stop the world ending, he was going to die fit, clean, well fed and engaged.

Desmond knew. He knew that the centrifugal force of despair is exacerbated by inertia. If you move, it can't getcha. As much. Or at all. It's why many doctors would prefer to prescribe gym memberships than anti-anxiety medication, if budgets allowed. And it's why clinical studies have found that exercise is as effective as therapy or prescriptions, when treating depression. It's harder for depression to hit a moving target.

And the ultimate moving-for-happiness activity of choice? For me, it is learning something new, whether it's how to use ink over a watercolour paint wash, or how to tumble-turn in the local leisure centre pool. Our brains love learning; remember the cascade of dopamine that is released (see page 192)?

Screens are the arch-enemy of ordinary joy

It's stating the bleedin' obvious, but when we're staring at screens, we're missing out on ordinary joy. I now know that my phone use is on a pulley system with my mental health. As my screen time goes up, my well-being goes down. They are inextricably, inconveniently connected.

If you're riveted by your iPad, you're not noticing that the cute two-year-old on the table over is hard-staring you, as if you're an enigma they want to crack. (I love impolite kid stares.) Instead, you're watching what the cast of *Made In Chelsea* (just me? Oh) are ~~selling~~ doing on Instagram. Instead of seeing the silhouette of Edinburgh Castle in the distance that tourists would exclaim over, you're looking at the view of a Maldives beach that a premiership footballer is admiring.

Instead of laughing about the teens engaged in a game of bin basketball with scrunched-up paper, you're laughing about what Kristen Wiig said on telly last night. Instead of appreciating that your six-year-old wants to have a 'litter picking party' (Real thing. Generation Z are already impressing me), you're appreciating the latest thing your political hero of choice (if you have one, these days it's slim pickings) has said.

I'm not in my actual life, when I'm looking at a screen. I'm someplace else. As are you. You're not with your friend at dinner, you're with the trolls on Twitter. You've been airlifted out of your life, and plunked into the bedroom of an influencer, or onto the rugby pitch, or into The White House.

And sometimes that's absolutely cool, since at times escapism is *dope* (particularly when it involves dragons; can I get a heckyeah from the *GoThroners*), but not all the dang time. Because that means we're living vicariously through other people's lives, rather than actually living our own.

What Madonna, or Freddie Flintoff, or Eckhart Tolle is doing right now may well be more interesting than what I'm doing, but 'Live your life, not theirs, Cath', is what I remind myself of now, over and over and over.

What you want vs what society wants for you

Our concern with what others think often drives our tireless pursuit of the extraordinary, when we would actually be quite content with *staying where we are*.

I read something that really stayed with me, in Bronnie Ware's *The Top Five*

---

* You can watch this on YouTube under 'Desmond – Make your own kind of music', if you're so inclined.

Regrets of the Dying. She reported that the topmost regret of those on their death bed was, 'I wish I'd had the courage to live a life true to myself, not the life others expected of me'. (Closely followed by 'I wish I hadn't worked so hard' and 'I wish I'd had the courage to express my feelings'.)

An excellent test as to whether something is truly worth pursuing, or doing, or getting, is if you would still chase it like the clatters, get stuck in, or buy it if you could never tell anyone.

Would you want that promotion, if it were an MI5-level secret? Would you get married, if there was no big party, ring or social acclaim attached? Would you move to that new house, if it were invisible? Would you want that luxury blender, if nobody else got to see it? This is a controversial one, but would you have children, even?

What we want, and what society wants us to do, often become blurred, indistinguishable, and need to be divided. I constantly have to un-plait the two in my brain, otherwise I find myself forgetting what I actually want, and trotting obediently down the path that is expected of me.

In a much-disputed John Lennon quote, he (apparently, who knows) said, 'When I was five years old, my mum always told me that happiness was the key to life. When I went to school, they asked me what I wanted to be when I grew up. I wrote down "happy". They told me I didn't understand the assignment and I told them they didn't understand life.' I mean, who really cares whether he said it or not, this quote is everything.

I very much doubt you or I will lie on our death beds and be transported by a showreel of 'extraordinary moments', such as the sky-diving, the view from the Space Needle or the dessert garnished with actual gold. We'll probably lie there and instead think of simple, homespun moments with our family and friends.

Outwitting the 'done' trapdoor in our brains

Remember the 'Dear me of a year ago'* letter that we talked about? This is one of the most transformative things I have learnt. Why? Because of the fantastically maddening Zeigarnik effect (page 92), whereby completed tasks fall out of a 'done' chute in our brains, which means we need to actively 'No! Don't lose that!' hang onto the many, many things we have achieved.

I'm an unmarried, sober, childfree non-homeowner about to turn 40.

---

* If you want even more well-being wallop, try a 'Dear me of three years ago' letter.

All of which looks bad on paper, says society, and yet, I'm happy as a damn clam. Because I'm always now reminding myself how far I've run on this inconvenient hedonic treadmill, rather than legging it after the next thing.

On a micro, daily level, I also include the things I've achieved that day on my gratitude list. It means I end the day exalting myself, rather than excoriating myself, even if all I've achieved is three things + breathing. You'll know if you have a child, a dog, or employees, that positive reinforcement is a more effective motivator than negative reinforcement, but we often forget to apply that rule to someone really important: ourselves.

Given we hedonically adapt financially too, and very quickly forget where we've clawed our way up from, I constantly remind myself of this fact. Just a few years ago, I was barely clearing five figures in my yearly salary, so I walked around the supermarket roughly totting things up in my head. I had to watch my money like a hawk eyeballing a mouse, because if I wasn't careful, that mouse would slink off, and I wouldn't have anything to eat, and I would have to call my parents AGAIN and ask for a loan AGAIN.

I knew I was lucky to be able to ask my parents in the first place, but it was an enormously stressful place to be. (If you are there right now, I see you, I salute you, and I *know* what you go through.)

So, now I don't forget my fortunate enoughness. I can sling things into the trolley without even thinking, 'Can I afford these fancy octagonal £2 cheese crackers?' I *can* afford them, and for that, I will never forget to feel grateful.

I now know to ignore my irrational, more-fixated brain, which is shouting 'Move it dipshit! Faster faster faster!', like the military bootcamp guy hollering at people in the park who are about to drown in their own sweat.

I am still miles behind most of my friends financially (and particularly property wise, given I don't own one) but *shrugs*. I now know money and property are not the fast lane to contentment, and I now definitely *don't* want to get to six figures, given I know about the 'high rollin' means high-happiness' myth.

My life/work balance (life is first, on purpose) is now my priority over money. Because once you have enough to live comfortably, I now know that money is like a cactus: best ignored.

Our brains will always bias the negatives

My brain is still negatively-biased…because I have one. The same is very likely true of yours too. When I was a week off my deadline for this book, I received an email from Apple saying that my MacBook Pro is one of the rogue older models whose battery is liable to overheat and catch fire, so I should stop using it immediately and return it to an Apple shop for maintenance.

I mean, this was at a point in my workload where even being separated from my laptop for *an hour* made me want to cry. Leaving it at the Apple shop for maintenance was simply unthinkable.

'Holy fuckin shittinhell!' went my brain's amygdala (the Chihuahua). 'Your laptop is about to spontaneously burst into blue flame!'

But now I know what I know, so I invited my prefrontal cortex (who is Gandhi, by the way) to step in and intervene. He reasoned that given I back up via iCloud, and also manually, *and* that my laptop has thus far never burst into flames, it was unlikely to in the next week. Ergo, I calmed the chuff down.

Like everything else that has been a personal odyssey of transformation for me mentally, this ability has been created by one simple thing. Learning everything I can about it. Learning why my brain flips out like this, which demystifies it, and thus removes its power over me.

That's how I learnt to stop drinking seven to eight bottles of wine a week and how to be happy sober, and also was how I learnt to be satisfied as a single, rather than feeling like a bisected panto pony.

So, I hope this book has enabled you too to be, 'I see you, I hear you, but I'm ignoring you,' towards your brain's negative bias. It's only trying to save your skin, but you can overwrite it with persistent positivity.

Yes, your laptop may be an urgent fire risk, or you may get mugged walking home late at night, and Chihuahuas do sometimes get eaten by seagulls (real news story I wish I could un-know), but the rational part of your brain knows that's highly unlikely to actually occur.

The core of the chore

Reminding ourselves of the core purpose of the chore, the desire at the root of the difficult, is transformative, says neuroscientist Dr Korb. 'We don't actually mind suffering per se, but we really do mind suffering for no reason.' So if you're having an awkward conversation with a partner, for instance, have in mind the point of it, such as: 'my partner is very important to me'. It's easier to have a difficult experience when the purpose of the pain is at the forefront of your mind.

For instance, these aren't remotely 'difficult' experiences, but I loathe hanging up wet clothes and I deep-sigh like a spoilt kid over plucking the leaves off herbs. I know. These are non-problems. I like having clean, crease-free clothes, and I love fresh herbs in my food, so I need to get over myself.

What's my alternative to doing these 'chores' myself? A laundry service wouldn't quite do the full job, and you can't buy fresh herbs minus the stems. So, paying a live-in maid? Well, she'd have to share my bed, given I have no spare room, which would be weird for us both. And I would have no disposable income for anything other than food. So. The maid and I would just sit in every night eating our food before going to my bed together, but at least we'd have fresh coriander sprinkled over it.

Therefore, I'll carry on doing these things myself. I concentrate on the grassy parsley smell, or how lucky I am to own a washing machine, and try to forget what a #middleclassnightmare I am currently enduring. (Please feel free to heckle me about my 'first world herb problems', should you ever meet me.)

Pleasure, interrupted

When I am in a pleasurable moment, I remember the revelation from page 21 about 'pleasure interrupted'. Eating a cookie or two at a time, rather than the full packet; watching a half hour of TV and then doing ten minutes of tidying; or interspersing DIY activities you enjoy (painting a wall, ahhh) with activities you don't (sanding furniture, uggg). The denial of the pleasure, the interruption of the enjoyable, actually enhances it. It feels outlandishly odd, at first, but it works.

Alternatively, when I'm in a less than pleasurable moment, I talk myself into wanting to be there. 'Happiness is not having what you want, but wanting what you have,' said a wise man, Rabbi Hyman Schachtel.

Nobody is going to wave a wand and transmute your breakdown-prone, slightly smelly car into a Venetian gondola. So – try wanting to be there. I find that if I replace, 'I don't want to be on this coach, I hate this coach, coaches suck, get me off this fecking coach!' with 'I want to be on this coach, because I want to get to where it is going', that creates a subtle, but profound mental shift.

The astronaut who fell in love

It's a totally unsubstantiated urban fable, but it also contains one of the most stunning sentiments I've ever heard*, so even if it is a myth, I don't care. Enter

---

* I first heard this story in the film, *Another Earth*, which is equally as gorgeous.

the story of the Russian cosmonaut.

The cosmonaut is orbiting the earth, alone, for almost a month, when this ticking starts. Tick, tick, tick. From beneath the dashboard. Of course, he tries to make it stop. He rips apart the control panel and tinkers around. Nothing makes the infernal sound stop.

After a few days of the ticking, he starts to feel that it will tick him into insanity, during his remaining 25 solitary days among the stars. So, he makes a mind-altering decision. To fall in love with the sound. To hear a metronome – and eventually, music – rather than an irksome ticking.

When you cannot change something, you can make the choice to fall in love with it instead. Whether it's your shower that's more watering can than tropical rainfall. Or the shopkeeper who is always incredibly rude to you, no matter how kind you are to him. (Happy people aren't mean, so he's fighting a battle you know nothing about.) Or balling a melee of 50-plus tiny, pastel children's socks.

This is how I apply the Russian cosmonaut story to real life. I'm the kind of sleeper who prefers absolute silence, and would wear a sound-cancelling motorcycle helmet to bed if I could sleep in it, so when I moved to a flat near a main road, I spent many nights listening to soundtracks of campfires crackling or hush-voiced bedtime stories, in order to try to eradicate the swoosh of cars and rumble of lorries.

Until I realized that the traffic actually sounds a lot like the ocean, and decided to fall in love with it instead. It worked. I would still choose silence, but given I've re-framed the cars as a mechanical lullaby, I can now sleep through them.

We can become besotted with the bland, or make the sensationally dull sublime. Enter the absolute ballers of ordinary joy – 'The Dull Men's Club'. Founded in the late eighties in NYC, it's now based in Britain, and the 5,000 or so members get together to 'celebrate the ordinary'. One of their straplines is 'Born to be mild'. Grrrr.

There's Kevin, who is the president of the UK's roundabout appreciation society (his nickname is 'Lord of the Rings'), and Steve, who has 20,000 milk bottles from around the globe (since you ask, no, he doesn't like milk), or Amanda (seems women are allowed in, thankfully), who spontaneously follows brown road signs to tourist attractions such as castles, theme parks and viewpoints.

Amanda's tourist-sign following is something I have started doing too, and highly recommend. I am originally from the Antrim Coast, and only just recently visited the Giant's Causeway and the Dark Hedges, both of which are under an hour's drive from my family's home village. Why did it take me nearly 40 years to get there? We so often forget to appreciate, or even visit, that which is on our very doorstep.

Other planets cannot be as beautiful

In my apricot'n'brown seventies kitchen, I have a plate by the illustrator Rob Ryan on display which reminds me of my biggest-ever gratitude.

It says, 'Other planets cannot be as beautiful as this one'. And it's true. Even when they CGI-imagine other planets, as in *Avatar*, it's still not a patch on planet earth. We're lucky to live here*. And yet we – I – forget that constantly. Because it's just *there*, a given, like gravity or the sun.

If you're going to give gratitudes a whirl, and if you're more scientifically-inclined than woo-woo (snap – me too) then maybe try to see the act of recording the positives as simply evening out the neuroscientific fact of your brain's negative bias.

Remember the five-to-one ratio weighting, from page 116? Yeah, that. Given the bad is bigger, we need to coax our prefrontal cortex into collecting the good, wherever we can. As the 'Father of American Psychology' William James once said, 'Only those items which I notice shape my mind'.

Also, as preposterous as it may seem to be writing about the joke you shared with a neighbour, or the really nice sandwich you just made, re-living these moments has unexpected clout a month, or a year down the line.

An elegantly executed 2014 study asked people to create time capsules filled with quotidian details such as the last party they attended, a recent conversation, so on, so boring. They discovered that, contrary to their expectations, the participants *loved* combing back over these seemingly unmemorable moments. 'We found that people are particularly likely to underestimate the pleasure of rediscovering ordinary, mundane experiences, as opposed to extraordinary experiences,' the authors wrote. Awooga! I rest my case.

As for where I am mentally these days, I won't use the word 'blessed', because it offends the natural-born pessimist in me. But I will say this: I'm (now) grateful. I wasn't for a long time. Now, when I'm trying to coax myself into slumber, I'm not musing on a magical kingdom far, far away where all my

---

* Also, we wouldn't be able to actually breathe on the other planets in our solar system, so y'know, there's that too. Yay for breathing!

extraordinary dreams have come true; I'm thinking on what I already have. What has already happened.

I now feel lucky to live here, on my scruffy street, in my modest flat, in my unremarkable life, and in my average skin. I'm not about to turn into Taylor Swift any time soon, so accepting what is – and becoming smitten with my ordinary life – is the biggest favour I could ever extend to myself. I don't need an upgrade, and nor do you.

As for my ordinary body and inexorable age, my best possible bottom may indeed be behind me as I head into the hinterland of midlife, but it's bloody lovely to know that my best possible mental health is most likely ahead of me (page 7).

The wall-to-wall ordinary upon which we live can be just as, if not *more* satisfying. It doesn't necessarily need ripping up and replacing. If we think of our lives as a living room, the extraordinary is that tiny but expensive ornament in the corner; while the ordinary is *the rest of it*.

So, let's enchant the rest of it, shall we? We have nothing to lose, other than our disenchantment.

THE COTTAGE

I'll leave you with this story.

When I was a kid, we used to go to this cottage in Donegal which was halfway up a mountain. We literally had to abandon the car a half-mile away, and tackle the final furlong, a hardscrabble path, laden down like packhorses.

'The Cottage' as we used to call it, has near-mythic status in my brain. But it was about as far from a five-star hotel as you can possibly get, with the possible exception of a camping holiday. A low, hunched, heavy-lidded stone creature, it was utterly bereft of any modern conveniences.

There was no running water, so we collected spring water and boiled it. Thus there were no showers, so bathing was either in a tin bath beside the fire in the winter, or a brief shrieking run and splish into the Coca-Cola-brown waterfall, flanked with emerald moss.

There was no electricity, so TV was a distant memory, meaning we had to actually talk to one another, play Gin Rummy, and read Famous Five books by candlelight. There was no central heating, so we slogged up to the top of the mountain to slice turf from it to burn.

A 'big day out' was a drive to the local pub, where ancient men would grumble expletives at each other from bar stools, and we would be treated to a Football Special and some Tayto crisps.

Or, if the shy Irish sun showed its face, we would drive to one of those lonely, magnificent Irish beaches that could rival a Greek island's best offering. And drive back with that salty, sun-toasted feeling running through our core like 'Donegal' through a stick of pink rock; which felt all the more sweet for being rare.

If you wanted to see views, you clambered up the mountain in muddy wellies. Without Nintendo Switches to hand us *Tomb Raider*-esque storylines, my brother and I made up our own, whereby we were King and Queen of our kingdom of sheep.

All the pleasure we had at The Cottage was made all the more exquisite by way of contrast. Get cold cutting turf; get warm burning turf. Work up hunger and thirst walking miles, slake it with Irish stew. Wear self out dragging body out of potentially deadly bog; rest self on utilitarian (but happily non-lethal) bunkbeds.

It was heavenly. And I don't rhapsodize this way about the bling hotels I've stayed at. I don't remember their names, I don't remember exactly where they were, I don't think of them often, and I don't long to be teleported back there. The trophy holidays simply don't compare.

The Cottage made me feel something far more ordinary, but infinitely more joyful.

SOURCES

INTRODUCTION

Ordinary definition, synonyms and antonyms: edited, abridged version of Lexico entry; Oxford dictionaries.

Three in ten Brits 'happy with their lives': Survey of 2,000 people, cited in Rose Troup Buchanan, 'Just three in ten Brits are happy with their lives', published on *The Independent* online, 23 January 2015.

One in six of us experiences a bout of anxiety or depression at least once a week: Statistic cited on mind.org.uk website under 'Mental health facts and statistics', at time of research (June 2019).

We spend on average five years of our life bored: OnePoll study commissioned by The British Heart Foundation cited in article by Rob Knight, '2,000 adults found we succumb to boredom twice a day', *The Independent*, published online, 10 September 2018.

Rates of depression worldwide increased by 18 per cent between 2005 and 2015: World Health Organisation, 'Mental health in the workplace', published online, 10 October 2017.

The happiest age group are those between 70 and 74 years old, data collated in 2012 and 2017: See Figure 3c graph, Office for National Statistics (ONS), 'Well-being, Personal well-being in the UK, October 2016 to September 2017', published online by the ONS, 26 February 2018.

SURVIVAL OF THE MOST NEGATIVE

Dr John Cacioppo dubbed one of the founding fathers of social neuroscience in his *New York Times* obituary, published 26 March 2018.

Brain reacts more strongly to negative bias than positive: TA Ito, JT Larsen, NK Smith and JT Cacioppo, 'Negative information weighs more heavily on the brain: The negativity bias in evaluative categorizations', published in the *Journal of Personality and Social Psychology,* 1998.

We find angry faces faster due to the 'anger superiority effect': CH Hansen et al. 'Finding the face in the crowd: An anger superiority effect', published in the *Journal of Personality and Social Psychology*, 1988.

THE HEDONIC TREADMILL

Ed Diener on how spending more of our income leads to lower happiness: Ed Diener and Robert Biswas-Diener, 'Will Money Increase Subjective Well-Being?', published in *Social Indicators Research*, 57, 2002.

Beyond the Hedonic Treadmill paper: Ed Diener, Richard E Lucas, Christie N Scollon, 'Beyond the hedonic treadmill: revising the adaptation theory of well-being', published in *American Psychologist*, 61, 2006.

SATISFICERS VS MAXIMIZERS

Professor Paul Dolan's quotes on brain scans, maximizing/satisficing, and salary: Paul Dolan, *Happy Ever After: escaping the myth of the perfect life*, pages xi, 1 and 6 respectively, Penguin Random House, 2019.

Steve Jobs' wife Laurene quote, taken from an interview with her which appeared in: *Steve Jobs*, Walter Isaacson, Simon & Schuster, 2011.

Simon Pegg sandwiches quote: cited from an interview with Elizabeth Day, *How to Fail: Everything I've ever learned from things going wrong*, Fourth estate, 2019.

I LOCATE THE EXACTITUDE OF GRATITUDE

40 per cent of happiness is intentional activity, plus re-playing blessings lessens their impact: S Lyubomirsky, KM Sheldon and D Schkade, 'Pursuing Happiness: The Architecture of Sustainable Change', published in the *Review of General Psychology*, volume 9, 2005.

University of Pennsylvania gratitude letter study: Martin Seligman, Tracy Steen, Nansook Park, Christopher Peterson, 'Positive Psychology Progress: Empirical Validation of Interventions', published in *The American Psychologist*, July 2005.

WHY EXTRA STUFF MEANS EXTRA 'SHOULDS'

51 per cent of Brits didn't read a book in 2018: Kantar Media, 2019.

A NON-INSTAGRAM-READY HOME

Ed Diener reports that we have on average six items on our wish-list (rounded down from the 6.3 cited) and that 47 per cent of us desire a bigger and better living space: Ed Diener and Robert Biswas-Diener, 'Will Money Increase Subjective Well-Being?', published in *Social Indicators Research,* volume 57, 2002.

DEAR GENERATION RENT

London most expensive city in Europe to rent: 2019 research from Employment Conditions Abroad, which compared the average costs of renting in 279 cities.

48 per cent year-on-year wealth growth needed for Millennials to catch up with baby boomers: cited in the Financial Conduct Authority's paper, 'Intergenerational Differences', May 2019.

ANXIETY IS SPECTACULARLY NORMAL

Hangxiety is worse in those who are 'shy': B. Marsh, M. Carlyle et al, 'Shyness, alcohol use disorders and 'hangxiety': A naturalistic study of social drinkers', published in *Personality and Individual Differences,* volume 139, 2018.

AN ODE TO WHERE THE WILD THINGS ARE

Essex forest walk 88 per cent, versus shopping centre at 44.5 per cent: (rounded up in copy to 45) cited in a report published by Mind in 2007 entitled 'Ecotherapy: the green agenda for mental health', accessed online through mind.org.uk

MID-RANGE SELF-ESTEEM

Nicholas Emler quotes: Nicholas Emler, *Self-esteem: the costs and causes of low self-worth*, York: York Publishing Services Ltd, 2001.

AN ODE TO LIE-INS

Arianna Huffington quotes and reported details of Marissa Mayer's, Richard Branson's and Donald Trump's sleep patterns: cited in Emine Saner, 'Arianna Huffington on why she wants you to sleep in her bed', published on the *Guardian* online, 6 April 2016.

Larks and owls are genetically determined: Y Hu, A Shmygelska, D Tran, N Eriksson, JT Tung and DA Hinds, 'GWAS of 89,283 individuals identifies genetic variants associated with self-reporting on being a morning person', published in *Nature Communications*, 2001.

NOBODY GETS 100 PER CENT GOOD REVIEWS

Matt Haig on how he deals with bad reviews: cited in Matt Haig, *Notes on a Nervous Planet*, Canongate, 2018.

Reviews on Gandhi and Michelle Obama cited: from public reviews on amazon.co.uk.

Dog inoculates against the lower mental well-being of social exclusion; Nilüfer Aydin, Joachim Krueger et al, 'Man's best friend: How the presence of a dog reduces mental distress after social exclusion', published in the *Journal of Experimental Social Psychology*, January 2012.

AN ODE TO CLEANING

2007 Harvard study on 84 hotel maids: Alia J Crum and Ellen J Langer, 'Mind-set matters: Exercise and the placebo effect', published in *Psychological Science* volume 18, no 2, 2007.

WE ARE NOT UNFLAPPABLE ANDROIDS

One of many studies that show naming emotions helps: Matthew D Lieberman, Naomi I Eisenberger et al, *Putting Feelings Into Words,* Psychological Science, volume 18, 2007.

FBI hostage negotiaters, plus more on naming emotions: Michael J McMains, C Wayman, *Crisis Negotiations: managing critical incidents and hostage situations in law enforcement and corrections*, Routledge, 2010.

WHEN SUNNY-SIDE-UP PSYCHOLOGY GOES TOO FAR

One of many studies that show suppressing emotions doesn't work: J J Gross and RW Levenson, 'Hiding Feelings: The Acute Effects of Inhibiting Negative and Positive Emotion', published in the *Journal of Abnormal Psychology*, volume 106, 1997.

Faking happiness at work is linked to heavier drinking afterward: AA Grandey et al 'When are fakers also drinkers? A self-control view of emotional labor and alcohol consumption among US service workers', published in the *Journal of Occupational Health Psychology,* 4 March 2019.

AN ODE TO NEVER GETTING ALL YOUR TO-DOS DONE

41 per cent of our to-do lists remain undone: iDoneThis app data.

To-do lists help people fall asleep more quickly: MK Scullin, ML Krueger, HK Ballard, N Pruett and DL Bliwise, 'The effects of bedtime writing on difficulty falling asleep: A polysomnographic study comparing to-do lists and completed activity lists'. Published in the *Journal of Experimental Psychology: General,* January 2018.

YOUR 'LOGICAL' FAMILY

Robin Dunbar quotes on friends: Aylin Woodward, 'With a little help from my friends', published in the *Scientific American* online, 1 May 2017.

SHRINKING OUR SKYSCRAPER-TALL EXPECTATIONS OF RELATIONSHIPS

2014 study on more than 100 couples: Lydia Emery, Amy Muise, Emily Dix, Benjamin Le, 'Can You Tell that I'm in a Relationship? Attachment and Relationship Visibility on Facebook', published in the *Personality & Social Psychology Bulletin*, September 2014.

IN PURSUIT OF THE SEX-TRAORDINARY

Data on 26,000 American couples and frequency of sex: Jean M Twenge, Ryne A Sherman, Brooke E Wells, 'Declines in Sexual Frequency among American Adults, 1989–2014', published in the *Archives of Sexual Behavior*, November 2018.

A BUDGET WEDDING AND WHY IT MEANS
YOU'RE LESS LIKELY TO DIVORCE

Those who spend more on their weddings are more likely to divorce: A Francis-Tan and HM Mislon, 'A Diamond is Forever' and Other Fairy Tales: the relationship between wedding expenses and marriage duration', published online at *SSRN papers*, volume 27, September 2014.

Professor Hugo Mialon quotes: cited in Chelsea Ritschel, 'Couples who spend more on their weddings are more likely to divorce, study finds', published on *The Independent* online, 6 July 2018.

Rewritten wedding vows and Brad Pitt quote: 'Some Seek Alternatives to 'til death do us part', Fox News online, 29 July 2005.

Jennifer Aniston marriages were a success quote: *Elle* magazine quote cited in Ree Hines article, 'Jennifer Aniston opens up about her "very successful" past marriages', published on *USA Today* online, 7 December 2018.

BREAK-UPS ARE MORE COMMON THAN NOT

Five-to-one ratio needed for couples to be happy: John Gottman, James Coan, Sybil Carrere and Catherine Swanson, 'Predicting Marital Happiness and Stability from Newlywed Interactions', published in the *Journal of Marriage and Family*, volume 60, no 1, February 1998.

THE MYTH THAT SINGLE IS AN UNDERORDINARY EXISTENCE

Paul Dolan's quotes about the reaction to his viral *Guardian* article about single, childfree women: Paul Dolan, 'Singled out: why can't we believe unmarried, childless women are happy?', published on the *Guardian* online, 4 June 2019.

Study of 22 countries shows the childfree are happier than those with children in countries such as the UK, USA and Australia: Jennifer Glass, Robin W Simon, Matthew A Anderson, 'Parenthood and Happiness: Effects of Work–Family Reconciliation Policies in 22 OECD Countries', 2016.

Professor Paul Dolan's quotes on brain scans, maximizing/satisficing and salary: Paul Dolan, *Happy Ever After: escaping the myth of the perfect life*, pages xi, 1 and 6 respectively, Penguin Random House, 2019.

JETTISONING 'PRESENTEEISM'

Seven of the top ten most productive countries work the least: OECD table and data from 2015, cited and reprinted in David Johnson, 'These are the most productive countries in the world', published in *Time* online, 4 January 2017.

A third of British people don't take their annual leave, on average losing four days of holiday a year: British Airways 2017 survey of 2,000 people, cited in Moya Sarner, 'The truth about why we don't use all our annual holiday leave', published on the *Guardian* online, 16 January 2018.

Daimler auto-delete while on holiday: reported by Chris Bryant, 'Auf Wiedersehen, Post', published on the *Financial Times* online, 13 August 2014.

AN ODE TO NOT DRIVING

Comments on 'peak car' and stats on driving licences by age group: Department of Transport research, 2018.

WHY BIG EARNING DOESN'T MEAN BIG HAPPINESS

Ed Diener cites studies that show rising wages correlate with higher divorce rates and stress, plus lower enjoyment of small activities: Ed Diener and Robert Biswas-Diener, 'Will Money Increase Subjective Well-Being?', published in *Social Indicators Research*, 57, 2002.

People who are happy earn higher incomes than those who are not happy: E Diener and MEP Seligman, 'Beyond Money: Toward an Economy of Well-Being', published in the *American Psychological Society*, volume 5, 2014.

Lottery winners compared to accident survivors: P Brickman, D Coates and R Janoff-Bulman, 'Lottery winners and accident victims: Is happiness relative?', published in the *Journal of Personality and Social Psychology*, volume 36, 1978.

Happiness scale compared to wealth index: Wealth index from Credit Suisse (2018). Happiness scale from LSE 'World Happiness Report', 2016–2018.

Complaining about being busy increases in line with income: D Hasermesh and J Lee, 'Stressed Out on Four Continents: Time Crunch or Yuppie Kvetch?', published by the Institute of Labor Economics, 2005.

Professor Paul Dolan's quotes on brain scans, maximizing/satisficing and salary: Paul Dolan, *Happy Ever After: escaping the myth of the perfect life*, pages xi, 1 and 6 respectively, Penguin Random House, 2019.

Gallup study finds emotional well-being plateaus at $75,000, 450K people asked: D Kaheman and A Reaton, 'High income improves evaluation of life but not emotional well-being'. *Proceedings of the National Academy of Sciences of the United States of America*, 2010.

Extraordinary experiences produce a comedown: Gus Cooney, Daniel T Gilbert, Timothy D Wilson, 'The Unforeseen Costs of Extraordinary Experience', published in *Psychological Science*, October 2014.

AN ODE TO SAVINGS

One in four have no savings, plus average savings amount of £4000: 2018 poll of 2620 Brits by Skipton Building Society.

Root of thrift: taken from the Online Etymology Dictionary.

BUSY AS A BADGE OF HONOUR

UCL study shows text and email ding your IQ by ten points, double the four-point drop seen in marijuana use: G Wilson, 'Text and Email reduces IQ more than cannabis', commissioned by the IT firm Hewlett Packard for TNS research, 25 April 2005.

AN ODE TO COMMON-OR-GARDEN PROCRASTINATING

One in five of us is a chronic procrastinator: cited in Heather Murphy, 'What we finally got around to learning at the Procrastination Research Conference', published on *The New York Times* online, 21 July 2017.

I WANT TO BE AN 'INFLUENCER'

2018 study shows more time on Instagram leads to higher levels of anxiety and depression: M Sherlock and DL Wagscott, 'Exploring the relationship between frequency of Instagram use, exposure to idealised images and psychological well-being in women'. Published in the *Psychology of Popular Media Culture*, 2018.

People who spend more time on Facebook liking, clicking and updating status, have a decrease in mental health: B Holly, N Shakya, A Christakis, 'Association of Facebook Use With Compromised Well-Being: A Longitudinal Study' published in the *American Journal of Epidemiology*, volume 185, issue 3, 1 February 2017.

Photo-impairment effect, study on art galleries: Linda A Henkel, 'Point-and-Shoot Memories: The Influence of Taking Photos on Memory for a Museum Tour', published in *Psychological Science*, December 2013.

AN ODE TO MILLENNIALS

Bret Easton Ellis, described as it appeared in the magazine: Decca Aitkenhead, 'American Psycho author Bret Easton Ellis on why he hates millennials', online version of the headline, *The Times* online, 21 April 2019.

Millennial men just as likely to call themselves a 'feminist' as Millennial women, and nine in ten Millennials believe in gender equality: Plan International UK survey, published 7 March 2017.

IN DEFENCE OF BEING AVERAGELY INFORMED

Dr Graham Davey quotes: Dr Graham Davey, 'The psychological effects of TV news', published on *Psychology Today* online, 19 June 2012.

Rough sleeping has risen 134 per cent since 2010: figures cited in 'Homelessness in England a 'national crisis' say MPs', published on BBC News online, 20 December 2017.

Homelessness in Britain figures: National Audit Office report, 'Homelessness', published 13 September 2017.

AN ODE TO BOOKS

We retain information better when we read on paper, rather than a screen: Lauren M Singer and Patricia A Alexander, 'Reading Across Mediums: Effects of Reading Digital and Print Texts on Comprehension and Calibration', published in *The Journal of Experimental Education*, March 2016.

AN ODE TO WHODUNNITS

Scott Bonn quote: from piece by Scott Bonn, 'Why we are drawn to true-crime shows', published on *Time* online, 8 January 2016.

Dr Amanda Ellison quote: from piece by Dr Amanda Ellison, 'Why watching TV crime dramas is good for your brain', published on *The Telegraph* online, 28 January 2015.

RE-DISCOVERING NINETIES AVAILABILITY

Mobile phone beats clock as most hated invention: 'Lemelsom-MIT Invention Index Study' finding in article by *MIT News*, published online, 21st January 2004.

Athena Chavarrion, Chris Anderson and Tim Cook quotes: Nellie Bowles, 'A dark consensus about screens and kids begins to emerge in Silicon Valley', published in the *New York Times* online, 26 October 2018.

Danish study on Facebook: conducted on 1,095 participants in 2015 by the Happiness Research Institute based in Copenhagen.

University of Texas phone presence study: Adrian F Ward, Kristen Duke, Ayelet Gneezy and Maarten W Bos at the University of Texas, 'Brain Drain: The Mere Presence of One's Own Smartphone Reduces Available Cognitive Capacity', published in the *Journal of the Association for Consumer Research,* volume 2, April 2017.

23 minutes, 15 seconds to recover from an electronic interruption: G Mark, D Gudith, and U Klocke, 'The Cost of Interrupted Work: More Speed and Stress', published by the University of California, Irvine.

Interruptions, or expectations of an interruption, creates a 20 per cent dumbing down: study commissioned by *The New York Times* and carried out by Alessandro Acquisti, a professor of information technology, and the psychologist Eyal Peer at Carnegie Mellon. Results cited in Bob Sullivan and Hugh Thompson, 'Brain, Interrupted', published on *The New York Times* online, 3 May 2013.

Zadie Smith quote from: 'I have a very messy and chaotic mind', published in *The Observer* magazine, 21 January 2018.

AN ODE TO LEARNING HOW TO BAKE A CAKE

Learning new things releases natural opium-like substances into brain: Irving Biederman,'"Thirst for knowledge" may be opium craving', published in *American Scientist*, 20 June 2006.

THE DIMINISHING RETURNS OF TV

Those who cap their TV use at two hours live 1.4 years longer, and over two-thirds of us watch more than two hours of TV a day: British study cited in article by Stephen Adams, 'Limit TV watching to 2 hours to live longer, say scientists', published in *The Telegraph* online, 10 July 2012.

More than 14 hours of TV a week linked to higher BMI and more depression: Abby C King et al, 'Identifying Subgroups of US Adults at Risk for Prolonged Television Viewing to Inform Program Development' published in the *American Journal of Preventive Medicine*, volume 38, January 2010.

AN ODE TO BOREDOM

Three-quarters of British children spend less time outside than prison inmates, they spend twice as much time on screens than outside, one in nine has not been to a natural environment in past year: Two-year study by Natural England, 'Monitor of Engagement with the Natural Environment pilot study: visits to the natural environment by children', published February 2016.

ON MEDIOCRE YET EXQUISITE CREATIVITY

Justin Rhodes quote: cited in 'Why is it that I seem to think better when I walk or exercise?', published in *Scientific American Mind*, July 2013.

IN PRAISE OF AVERAGE ATTRACTIVENESS

Our partners think we're more attractive than strangers do: V Swami, S Inamdar, S Stieger, IW Nader, J Pietschnig, US Tran and M Voracek, 'A dark side of positive illusions? Associations between the love-is-blind bias and the experience of jealousy', published in *Personality and Individual Differences*, 2012.

Altruism is attractive: D Moore, S Wigby, S English, S Wong, T Székely and F Harrison, 'Selflessness is sexy: reported helping behaviour increases desirability of men and women as long-term sexual partners'. Published in *BMC Evolutionary Biology*, volume 13, 2013.

Study on female body dissatisfaction, the skinny myth and attractive female body weight in 26 countries: V Swami et al, 'The attractive female body weight and female body dissatisfaction in 26 countries across 10 world regions: results of the international body project I', published in the *Personality & Social Psychology Bulletin*, volume 36, March 2010.

Link between beauty and shorter relationships: Christine Ma-Kellams, Margaret C Wang, Hannah Cardiel, 'Attractiveness and relationship longevity: Beauty is not what it is cracked up to be', published by *Wiley Online Library*, 3 February 2017.

Elle article on nineties brows. Mariel Tyler and Justine Carreon, 'What 26 celebs would look like with '90s brows', published by *Elle* online, 22 March 2018.

AGEING LIKE WE ARE INTENDED TO

Seven in ten sexagenarians are happy with their body: B Tobin, 'Over a third of Brits are unhappy with their bodies', published online by YouGov, 21 July 2015.

HAVING A REGULAR-SIZED BODY

37 per cent of Brits unhappy with body, plus 74 per cent blame celeb culture for negative female body image: B Tobin, 'Over a third of Brits are unhappy with their bodies', published online by YouGov, 21 July 2015.

Study on female body dissatisfaction, the skinny myth and attractive female body weight in 26 countries: V Swami et al, 'The attractive female body weight and female body dissatisfaction in 26 countries across 10 world regions: results of the international body project I', published in the *Personality & Social Psychology Bulletin,* volume 36, March 2010.

Those who have breast enlargements plus higher suicide rates: BD Sarwer, 'The psychological aspects of cosmetic breast augmentation', published in *Plastic Reconstructive Surgery*, 2007.

Average weight and size of British women: 2017 information provided by lingerie brand Bluebella, based on analysis of data from the fashion industry, the British Bra Survey, the Office of National Statistics and the NHS.

Timothy Frayling quote: cited in 'What's the main cause of obesity', published in the *British Medical Journal* online, 10 September 2012.

Average female shoe sizes have risen from size 4 in the 1960s to size 6.5 now: cited in J Laurance, 'Why are our feet getting bigger', published in *The Independent*, 3 June 2014.

Four in ten of us unhappy with teeth appearance: A survey of 666 participants by Cosmetic Surgery Solicitors, 2018.

Only 18 per cent of women orgasm through penetration alone: Debby Herbenick, Tsung-Chieh Fu, Jennifer Arter, Stephanie Sanders and Brian Dodge, 'Women's Experiences With Genital Touching, Sexual Pleasure, and Orgasm: Results From a US Probability Sample of Women Ages 18 to 94', published in the *Journal of Sex & Marital Therapy*, 9 August 2017.

AN ODE TO MIDLIFE

Happier at 40 than 18: Nancy Fang, Harvey Krahn, Matthew Johnson and Margie Lachman, 'Up, Not Down: The Age Curve in Happiness from Early Adulthood to Midlife In Two Longitudinal Studies' published in *Developmental Psychology* online, 7 September 2015.

Life expectancy calculator: 'What is my life expectancy? And how might it change?', published on the Office of National Statistics website, 1 December 2017. URL: https://www.ons.gov.uk/peoplepopulationandcommunity/healthandsocialcare/healthandlifeexpectancies/articles/whatismylifeexpectancyandhowmightitchange/2017-12-01

AN ODE TO SHOWERS

Hannah Jane Parkinson quote: Hannah Jane Parkinson, 'The joy of small things', *Guardian Weekend* magazine, page 65, 22 June 2019. Can also be accessed online under the headline, 'As I integrated back into regular life, brushing my teeth helped heal my mind'.

AN ODE TO MASSAGES

Massages increase serotonin by 28 per cent and decrease cortisol by 31 per cent: T Field, M Hernandez-Reif, M Diego, S Schanberg, C Kuhn, 'Cortisol decreases and serotonin and dopamine increase following massage therapy', published by the *International Journal of Neuroscience*, October 2005.

IN DEFENCE OF THE BOG-STANDARD WORK OUT

A fifth of those who own exercise bikes have only used it once. NOP poll in 2003 for St Ivel Gold.

Hannah Rice expensive trainer research: cited by Professor Vybarr Cregan-Reid in *Primate Change: how the world we made is remaking us*, page 209, Cassell, 2018.

MY MANIFESTO FOR NEVER LOSING ORDINARY JOY

2014 time capsule study showing we underestimate the power of recalling the ordinary: Ting Zhang, Tami Kim, Alison Wood Brooks, Francesca Gino, Michael I Norton. 'A "Present" for the Future: the unexpected value of rediscovery', published in *Psychological Science*, August 2014.

The top three regrets of the dying: Ware, B. *The Top Five Regrets of the Dying: A life transformed by the dearly departing,* Hay House, London, 2012.

Clinical studies show exercise is as effective as therapy or prescriptions: GM Cooney et al, 'Exercise for Depression', published in the *Cochrane Database of Systematic Reviews*, September 2013.

Dull Men's Club info: taken from interview/video made with Grover Click, one of the founders of the DMC, entitled 'The Simple Joys of the Dull Men's Club', published on YouTube by Great Big Story, 27 June 2017.

INDEX

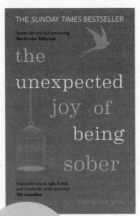

THE *SUNDAY TIMES* BESTSELLER

'hearty, shrewd and convincing'
The Sunday Telegraph

the
unexpected
joy of
being
sober

'Admirable honest, light, bubbly
and remarkably earth-annoying'
The Guardian

catherine gray

Going sober will make you happier, healthier, wealthier, slimmer and sexier. Despite all of these upsides, it's easier said than done. This inspirational, aspirational and highly relatable narrative champions the benefits of sobriety; combining the author's personal experience, factual reportage, contributions from experts and self-help advice.

Ever sworn off alcohol for a month and found yourself drinking by the 7th?

Think there's 'no point' in just one drink?

Welcome!

There are millions of us. 64 per cent of Brits want to drink less.

Also available as an ebook and audiobook

Catherine Gray was stuck in a hellish whirligig of Drink, Make horrible decisions, Hangover, Repeat. She had her fair share of 'drunk tank' jail cells and topless-in-a-hot-tub misadventures.

But this book goes beyond the binges and blackouts to deep-dive into uncharted territory: What happens after you quit drinking? This gripping, heart-breaking and witty book takes us down the rabbit-hole of an alternative reality. A life with zero hangovers, through sober weddings, sex, Christmases and break-ups.

In *The Unexpected Joy of Being Sober*, Catherine Gray shines a light on society's drink-pushing and talks to top neuroscientists and psychologists about why we drink, delving into the science behind what it does to our brains and bodies.

Much more than a tale from the netherworld of addicted drinking, this book is about the escape, and why a sober life can be more intoxicating than you ever imagined. Whether you're a hopelessly devoted drinker, merely sober-curious, or you've already ditched the drink, you will love this book.

THE SUNDAY TIMES BESTSELLING AUTHOR OF
THE UNEXPECTED JOY OF BEING SOBER

catherine gray

the
unexpected
joy of
being
sober
journal

A guided sobriety journal for motivation with prompts and reminders for Dry January, Sober Spring and beyond.

Also available as an ebook

PREFACE

Joan Didion, the super-cool American essayist, said, 'I don't know what I think until I write it down.' And that's how I was. I didn't know what I thought about drinking and sobriety, until I started writing about it.

I didn't intend to write a book. At all. If I time travelled right now back to 2013 and said, 'you're going to write a book about this one day' to the Drinking Me who was desperately trying to hide her empty bottles, shaking hands and shattered soul, she would have been horrified. She would have howled with shame.

For the first two years of writing this book, I absolutely intended to don the cloak of a pseudonym. I said to people, 'I can't talk about the shakes, about morning drinking, about promiscuity, about the wind-chime tinkle of tiny bottles in my bag, under my real name. HELL NO.'

But then I slowly realized that the people I admired the most in the sober-sphere are those who have chosen to step away from the shadows. Those who are fully 'out'. I was inspired by the 'I am not anonymous' movement*, a series of beautiful portraits of sober people. I realized that if I hid behind a fake name, I would effectively be saying that growing addicted to booze, or getting sober, are things to be ashamed of. Which they're really not.

I am no longer remotely ashamed. Unveiling some of these personal details puts me well out of my comfort zone, it's true. But, stigmas grow in the shadowlands. So, let's floodlight the sober movement. Alcohol is an addictive drug. There's no shame in not being able to use it moderately. You are not unusual if you can't stop at one or two. You're not broken. Or weak. You're actually the norm. Two-thirds of Brits are drinking more than they intend to.

We should be able to drop 'I don't drink' or 'I'm teetotal' or 'I'm taking a break from drinking' into conversation just as smoothly as we say 'I don't eat meat' or 'I'm a non-smoker' or 'I'm taking a break from dairy'. There shouldn't be any cringe around choosing to do something positive for your body and well-being.

---

*Check out www.iamnotanonymous.org. It's ace.

Our thinking about drinking, as a society, is wonky. Drinking is not inevitable. Or compulsory. We don't need to have a doctor's note to excuse us from swan-diving into wine. We don't have to be driving to say 'no ta'. And it's not just recovering alcoholics, like me, who can choose not to drink.

We have a collective shame around feeling like we're 'failing' at alcohol. We've been conditioned into that hangdog shame. We've been taught to hide away our struggles with alcohol. It's high time that changed. It's a moonshot goal, but I'm hoping this book will help re-brand and re-align how people see sobriety.

I hope this will start the 'I'm-drinking-too-much-and-I-don't-know-how-to-stop' conversation. Instead of sobriety being something a clutch of 'failed drinkers' have to do, it's something we all get to do. If we choose it.

Catherine

GETTING SMASHED IN SUBTERRANEAN SOHO

'Drinking steals happiness from tomorrow'
Unknown

The first time I got drunk I felt like I'd finally unzipped my 'wrong' skin and slipped into a slinky new one. One that felt ridiculously right. One without the spiky inhibitions. It was like taking off chainmail and slipping into a heavenly silk gown.

More than four in ten people who start drinking before the age of 15 will eventually become addicted to alcohol. I was 12 when I started. As an incredibly nervous kid, I began to believe that relief resided in bottles. That great stories were at the bottom of glasses. That booze was anaesthetic for my ever-present anxiety.

Before drinking, my life had felt terribly dull. I started out with the classy combo of drinking White Lightning cider in the car park of McDonald's. By the age of 13, I was clubbing up to three times a week. My best mate and I fell in with a crowd of 17-year-olds who dressed us up in their clothes, helped us with our make-up and snuck us into The Venue and The Dorchester in Wolverhampton.

I was an indie kid, a grebo, who burned incense until my room stank of sandalwood, pierced my nose with a tiny silver stud, hennaed my hair and completed the effect with Doc Marten's and tiny flowery dresses. I basically wanted to be Angela Chase in *My So-Called Life*.

Magazines were my obsession; an escape from my humdrum existence. Every Wednesday I would hotfoot it to the newsagents with 70p in my hand, to buy *Just Seventeen*, and then trip over myself as I walked to the bus-stop reading it. I read about Justine *Elastica* and Sonya *Echobelly* and Marijne *Salad* and Louise *Sleeper* running around Soho and Camden. I wanted to go join them but I lived in Dudley, a running joke of a backwater Black Country town. People literally laughed in my face when I said I lived in Dudley.

Life was too sharp, too painful, too real and too loud when I was sober. Drinking softened the edges and blurred the clarity. It turned an intimidating Andy Warhol pop-art world into a misty Monet watercolour. Sober, nightclub dancefloors were about as appealing as the Mad Max Thunderdome. Drunk, they were my domain. It made me party-ready when I was party-meh. But, it wasn't real. That me was not *me*.

Blackouts were commonplace right from the get-go. I thought everyone experienced lost hours of nights out – turns out they don't. I thought everyone felt jangly-nerved and ill-fitting until they'd had a drink – turns out they don't. I'd always felt like I was on the outside, looking into social situations, never quite able to fully shed my inhibitions and engage. Booze opened the door, beckoned me in from the cold and thrust me into the thick of the party.

I only attended about a quarter of my lectures at university and yet, I managed to somehow scrape a 2:1, like a magician summoning coins from their sleeve. I thought I was addicted to going out with my mates, but the truth was, when all of my uni friends vacated the town for the summer and I stayed on to work my bar job, I still drank just as hard. With any company I could find, including the dubious regulars at the pub. Are you a big drinker? Great! Let's get blitzed.

I wrote dozens of letters begging for work experience on magazines. I spent a year doing a dull job in marketing to save money. I finally got my toe through the door and after a year of hardscrabble interning at *Glamour* and *Cosmopolitan*, I was offered a junior role at the latter.

I land in Soho

I loved my job and worked dang hard. But, my job came with a catch. A catch that I regarded as a boon. My job gave me access to nightly parties. I could drink most nights for free, if I wanted to. I wanted to.

I made the louche underbelly of Soho my home, chasing the night right until the end. I learned where the secret subterranean speakeasy bar was, Trisha's, hidden behind a gleaming cornflower-blue residential door, and learned the code word to get in. Trisha's was cluttered with tat, it reeked of fags, the wallpaper was peeling and the wine was warm. It never closed though, so it was my nirvana.

I watched Amy Winehouse perform an impromptu gig in a scruffy cubby-hole of a jazz bar on Greek Street. As she sang, 'They tried to make me go to rehab, I said no, no, no' I sang along. 'She can barely stand,' my mate whispered to me. I shrugged. I thought she was cool.

I blagged my way into the VIP room of a spangled casino hotel by saying I was Delta Goodrem (if you squinted, and it was very dark, I could have been back then, just). My mate and I (he was supposedly Brian McFadden, her boyfriend at the time) shared the living-room-sized space of the VIP with Victoria Beckham and Gordon Ramsay. We danced with them to Britney. Until the barman kindly escorted us out. VB sent us a bottle of champagne as a consolation prize.

I hung out in a handsome '50s mahogany-panelled, cigar-scented member's bar, with a Mafia-esque vibe, where men with magnificent moustaches would have cradled brandy and struck business deals. As I was leaving one night, I saw Christian Slater. I bounced over and told him I'd loved him in *Pump Up the Volume*. He said, 'Hang on, don't go' and invited me to join him for a drink. He said he liked my name, and rolled it around on his tongue like a butter candy. Cath-er-ine Graaaay.

I stayed out until 6am doing karaoke with Johnny Vegas. That night, rather than going home, which was pointless, I napped in the ladies' toilet at the *Cosmopolitan* offices, where I worked, and tried to wash myself in the sink.

I smoked weed with Finley Quaye. Stephen Dorff invited me to a Girls Aloud gig. Marco Pierre White told me he loved me at the end of our interview and invited me to dine anytime at his restaurant for free, which I never got around to doing, because, well, drinking got in the way. Eating was cheating. I always went for drinks, not dinner, even a free Michelin-starred dinner. I judged people who left wine on the table as harshly as I judge people who leave dogs in hot cars.

I was flown to Washington, DC first class when I worked at *Glamour*, and put up in an elegant five-star hotel to interview Reese Witherspoon. The moment the interview was in the bag, I went to a pavement cafe amid the rainbow townhouses of Georgetown and sank wine after wine, telling myself I was 'experiencing' DC. (It makes me want to cry that I didn't actually explore that great city.) I was invited to the White House to meet Michelle Obama the next day (along with about 100 other people). Even though I was scrubbed and coiffed for my trip to The White House, my hangover was bone-deep. When Michelle looked at me, shook my hand and said 'hello', her forehead furrowed with concern. (Smart woman, Michelle.)

This was the dream, no? This was the kind of life everyone wanted. My friends kept telling me how jealous they were of my job. I worked my tail off during the day and shook my tailfeather at night. I took the odd night off and pounded my urge to drink into submission at the gym.

But inside, cracks were beginning to show. I lived in a state of perpetual alarm that I would be busted, for lying about fictitious food poisoning, or that my blackout tryst with my male co-worker would be revealed. Fear ate away at me like invisible termites inside the walls of a house. My very structure and foundations were beginning to falter.

The party road toll

The partying took its physical toll. Calling in sick to work became a regular occurrence. The hangovers that I saved my sick days for were the paralyzing ones. The times when I felt I literally could not move from my bed for the entire day. Or the times when I woke up wearing last night's clothes, on the other side of London from my flat, at 10am (which was often).

I was often cautioned about having too many sick days in work reviews by my managers. They would make embarrassed jokes about me perhaps needing to take more vitamins, or gently temper the criticism with praise on how great my work ethic was the rest of the time. In the big picture, I was getting away with it. I was promoted again and again.

Nonetheless, the words 'can I have a word with you?' or a jokey 'I have a bone to pick with you' could send me into a terrified spin. My post-spin strategy? Patching up my hungover face and charging out into London to do it all over again.

I suffered from Wishful Drinking. Tonight would be the night I cracked it. The night I would have two drinks in the pub, laugh with my friends and go home, rosy-faced and aglow with wine, to make a stir-fry and have an early night. Tomorrow would be the morning I would actually get up and go for the 7am run before work, rather than groaning and stabbing at the alarm to make it stop. Like the desert spring the dying man crawls towards endlessly, but never reaches, I was never able to locate that oasis.

My ideal 'tonight' and 'tomorrow' remained shimmering in the distance. The vegetables for the stir-fry always lost their will to live in my fridge. It was always the same last-orders outcome. The same dejected night bus, the same urgent scrabbling in the morning, standing in the shower willing the water to wash off my shame, the same bacon sandwich at my desk with a full-fat Coke.

I was scared to sit still. To stay in. To take a long hard look at myself. If I kept going out, kept drinking, kept running this-a-way and that-a-way, I wouldn't have to actually confront what I'd become. A fraud, beneath the sequined dress and make-up. A liar who didn't actually want to lie but kept finding herself in situations where the options were: a) get dumped by your boyfriend, b) lie. Or, a) get sacked, b) lie. Or, a) get kicked out of your house by your flatmate, b) lie. Lying was simply something I had to do to survive.

Sometimes I had to write down the lies to remember them accurately. I would rehearse them in a soft voice in my room before seeing the unfortunate recipient of the lie, like an actor running lines. The thing with lying to everyone, to varying degrees? No one ever truly knows you. Which is a really lonely place to live.

But I also felt indignant. Why did the universe keep curve-balling these impossible dilemmas and predicaments my way?! It wasn't fair. I truly could not see that booze was a villain, rather than a hero. I thought it was the pain-remover, rather than the source of the pain. And I couldn't see that I was complicit. I was happening to life; life wasn't just happening to hapless me. I was the architect of my own destruction every single time, along with my trusty sidekick, wine.

An unnamed dread spread inside me like an ink blot. My fear that something Godawful was about to happen became more and more urgent. The 'watched' feeling grew. I was convinced people were starting to notice. I felt like cornered quarry. The only thing that drowned the dread, that pulverized the paranoia, was more wine.

I start to lose more than my bag

Alcohol unlocked my true self, I thought. I was willing to pay for that luxury. Sober, I just felt *wrong*.

What I didn't know was how terribly high the price was going to be. It was going to cost me friends, familial love, many boyfriends, the respect of my colleagues and all of my self-esteem. It was going to place me in dangerous situations – scenarios in which it was amazing I wasn't killed.

The pace was glacial, over the next 21 years. The scary times were one in a hundred. Then they were one in ten. Then every other time. Then just every single time. But I'd long forgotten there was an alternative.

Addiction has an imperceptible grip, that tightens ever-so-gradually. Nobody wakes up one day and suddenly can't stop drinking. The progression is apparent to others perhaps, but mostly dismissed with quizzical glances. However, the person themselves is usually totally oblivious, because they are shrouded deep in denial. Deep, deep, deep in denial.

For me, addiction manifested itself in the breaking of hundreds of tiny rules. Tiny threads that tethered me to the ground snapped, one by one. The rules of Normal Drinking. I never thought I'd use my last grocery money to buy wine; until I did. I never thought I'd drink in the morning; until I did. And once you've broken a rule once, it becomes very easy to break it again. And again.

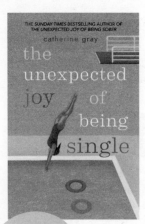

Also available as an ebook and audiobook

The highly anticipated follow-up to the *Sunday Times* bestseller *The Unexpected Joy of Being Sober.*

Having a secret single freak-out? Feeling the red, heart-shaped urgency intensify as the years roll on by?

Oh hi!

You're in the right place.

Over half of Brits aged 25–44 are now single. It's become the norm to remain solo until much later in life, given the average marriage ages of 35 (women) and 38 (men). Many of us are choosing never to marry at all.

But society, films, song lyrics and our parents are adamant that a happy ending has to be couple-shaped. That we're incomplete without an 'other half'*, like a bisected panto pony. Cue: single sorrow. Dating like it's a job. Spending half our lives waiting for somebody-we-fancy to text us back. Feeling haunted by the terms 'spinster' or 'confirmed bachelor'.

Catherine Gray took a whole year off dating to find single satisfaction. She lifted the lid on the reasons behind the global single revolution, explored the bizarre ways cultures single-shame, detached from 'all the good ones are gone!' panic and debunked the myth that married people are much happier.

Let's start the reverse brainwash, in order to locate – and luxuriate in – single happiness. Are you in?

*Spoiler: you're already whole

DRUNK ON LOVE

FEBRUARY, 2002

I've been on three dates with a charismatic, smooth, handsome older man –
Daniel. I've decided that Daniel is The Guy. Every day, at work, I keep half an
eye on my Nokia just in case its screen illuminates green and that wondrous little
envelope appears.

Every night, after I finish work, I go home and dial-up the internet. Bing,
bong, jjjjhhhhh, bong, bing, screeleebop, repeat.

Several minutes later, I am online. Booyah! I sit in front of my cathmermaid@
hotmail.com* homepage and click on my inbox. I am looking for a fix. My
substance. Relief from this constant craving. I am seeking an email from Daniel,
ideally arranging our next date. It's not there. Fucksticks.

I sit there, for the next two hours, constantly hitting 'refresh' on the computer.
Refresh, refresh, refresh. I really do.

When I get bored of my clicking, I read articles on vacuous websites with titles
such as 'How to get him hot for you', or '21 signs he's nuts about you' or 'Men on
their 19 date-dealbreakers'.

It's imperative I learn this poppycock, in order to bag Daniel. It's like I'm
revising for a test. OK, so I need to: play with my hair, not respond straight away,
be busy for the first two dates he suggests, reveal legs or cleavage but never both.
Check, check, check. Refresh, refresh, refresh.

I am totally oblivious to the fact that I'm obsessively clicking my inbox like
a rat in a laboratory cage. A rat with a button that dispenses a drug. I think my
behaviour is normal.

My behaviour was not normal. I was a raging love addict.

---

* *Millennials: this was back in the days when we all chose ludicrous email addresses. Think hotrod1979@
hotmail.com, lusciouslipslucy@yahoo.co.uk, beerpongbarry@outlook.com. Without ever thinking that these
would have to go on our CVs. We soon learned.*

INTRODUCTION

Monomania: Exaggerated or obsessive enthusiasm for or preoccupation with one thing. (Extracted from the *Oxford Dictionary*)
Oneomania: Exaggerated or obsessive enthusiasm with finding The One. (Extracted from my head)

I'm going to level with you. I am still a love addict. I can't claim to be fixed. Nope. Sorry. That would be a bare-faced lie.

Alas, I am still the woman who stares saucer-eyed at her text messages, watching her phone like a TV, breathlessly awaiting a reply when those tantalizing iPhone dots appear. I still have to gently slap myself around the face to stop the Yosemite Wedding fantasy (woodland-themed, if you must know, a little bit Narnian, with harpists and flutists, and I will wear...oh rats, there I go again *gentle slap*).

I still crush like a paper bag whenever a man I've only had two dates with, and barely know, who I've spent a grand total of (drum roll) seven hours with, ghosts me. I'm still that person. I'm not going to pretend otherwise.

However, I have managed to dial my oneomania down from urgent, hysterical, phone-stabbing, triple-messaging ('Are you OK? Have you had an accident?!'). It helped enormously that I took a whole year off dating, during which I didn't so much as hold a man's hand.

It helped that I read as much as I could about why love addiction happens, all of which I will impart to you. It helped that I stopped giving people the power to puff or deflate me. When I was chronically love-addicted, I was like an inflatable person; reliant on praise to pump me up and shrinking into a glum little heap when I felt rejected.

A spinster aged 33

My first love rock bottom came a couple of months before my final alcohol rock bottom. My dad, now sadly departed, started calling me a 'spinster' aged 33. And no, he wasn't yanking my chain. This was no 'just rattling your cage!' joke. He was being straight-down-the-line serious that I was a spinster, and what the devil was I gonna do about it.

This 'You're a spinster' conversation came about because of a visit we'd just made to my aunt and uncle. During which, the question 'So, any danger of you getting married, Catherine?' was asked. I explained that I'd just split up with a guy who hadn't been treating me well, who I'd lived with for a year, and that I felt good about the decision. My uncle frowned and said 'Well, you're not getting any younger,' which my dad guffawed at.

When we left, I turned to my dad, laughed nervously, and said 'They've started treating me like a spinster!' He said, matter-of-fact, unflinchingly, as was his way: 'Well, *you are a spinster.*' We then had a huge argument in the car, during which I cried, said I wasn't a spinster, and he shouted at me that I was a spinster. It was bizarre.

I was utterly distraught. Later that day, I went for a long run along the River Lagan, sat on a leafy riverbank and full-body-sobbed. Once I'd cried myself out, I tried to figure out why this had wounded me so much. I knew full well, rationally, that this was ridiculous fifties *Mad Men*-esque misogyny, and yet it had cut me deep. I explored my wound and found a thorn buried deep inside. A thorn of Failure. That was it. Huh. This was what had scored my side so brutally.

I felt like I'd failed as a woman, as a person, because I hadn't found my life partner yet. I felt unchosen, unwanted, left on the shelf. While also knowing, intellectually, that this was nonsense. I knew that I had just finished a toxic relationship and was, at the age of 33, a mere youngster in the grand scheme.

A friend once informed me that my photo albums resembled an ego-fluffing trophy room. The sort of room somebody despicable has hidden away, replete with stag antlers, rhino horns and stuffed leopards.

I recently looked back over said photo album, with a discerning eye. She was right. It was basically a Rolodex of my exes, with the odd mate thrown in. It was a display cabinet. Of men who had found me to be worthwhile. Now that I look at this album, it's highly creepy. My catalogue of kills. I really did define myself by the men I'd slept with.

But, d'you know what? I completely understand why I was the way I was. I don't judge my twentysomething self. I'd been taught that romantic relationships are *the most important thing*, over and over, through subliminal (or blatant) societal messaging. As have you.

Settle down, quick!

Here's the thing. We've been brainwashed into thinking that a happy-ever-after always involves finding a partner. The person. Our lobster. Our other half. How is it that, in the 21st century, getting married is still seen as a woman's greatest accomplishment? Is it my imagination, or is that undercurrent really there? (I think it's really there.) And, it's not just women who feel this intense pressure. Men feel it too.

Yet, despite this proposal press-gang, millions of us are increasingly choosing to stay single. The single population is growing at ten times the rate of the population in general. A typical British Millennial is expected to live alone, without a partner, for an average of 15 years.

The most recent data, collated by Mintel in their *Single Lifestyles* 2017 report, found that 51 per cent of Brits aged 25–44 are now single (including divorcees). Back in 2016, the Office for National Statistics reported that the single/divorced slice of the population was 35 per cent. Could that seriously be a jump of 16 per cent in one little year?

We're leaving marriage later and later. The Office for National Statistics released a report in 2018 that said, 'For marriages of opposite-sex couples, the average (mean) age for men marrying in 2015 was 37.5 years, while for women it was 35.1 years.'

In other words, the average bride was 35 years old, while the average groom was circa 38. This revelation triggered a slew of press headlines, such as 'Rise of the Older Bride: average age for women to walk down the aisle is now over 35.' Out of these 2015 marriages, 75 per cent of the men and 76 per cent of the women were marrying for the first time. Six in ten brides were over 30.

In 1970, average marriage ages were 27 for men and 25 for women. So, compared to 1970, men are getting married 11 years later, while women are getting married 10 years later. Astounding, huh?

What's more, 42 per cent of marriages end in divorce. Meaning that almost half of those who walk hopefully and beaming down the aisle, wind up suddenly single later in life.

Single is now the norm

Before I dug up this data showing that singles have now tipped over into becoming the majority, I wrote reams of cool stuff about norm-subverting, which then had to hit the cutting room floor, once I found out that *we are now the norm*. I didn't know that. Did you?

However, even though it *is* that way, it doesn't *feel* that way. It still feels rebellious, like trend-bucking, to be single later in life. Why? Because we are still living in the shadow of the nuclear-shaped family and groaning under the weight of our parents' expectations.

We'll talk more about this later, but during the raising and adulting of the Baby Boomer generation, there was an almighty marriage spike, which is likely why our parents are so perplexed that we're not married *like they were* by our age. (If you're aged 25–50, you're most likely the offspring of Baby Boomers.)

Our parents and the media have taught us to fear being single. I know this fear, intimately. It's why I was never single in my twenties, and instead swung from boyfriend to boyfriend. I thought *any* relationship, no matter how toxic, was better than none. When I wasn't with someone I felt flat and dark, like a pitch-black room that waits for someone to come along, flick on the light, and animate it once more. And ironically, given the paramount importance I awarded the preservation of relationships, I was a human wrecking ball. I snooped, cheated, started arguments, all that fun stuff. I would break up with people to push a lever for more attention.

In recent years, I've managed to stop all of that. I don't stay in unhealthy relationships, I'm no longer frightened of being single, I can date without losing my marbles, and I've now learned to luxuriate in my singleness, rather than look longingly at couples thinking, 'I want that. Why don't I have that?'

As I say, I'm not *cured* of love addiction. It's still running around inside me, growling for sustenance. But I've learned how to live with it. How to tame it, leash it, re-train it, even stroke it. And I'm now genuinely happy as a single.

Working on my love addiction has led to me now feeling free of the need to be coupled. In my twenties I was single for a grand total of six months (which were basically spent interviewing potential new boyfriends) and in the past five years I've been single for three-and-a-half *years*. That's a rise from 5 per cent singleness in my twenties, to 70 per cent in the past five years.

Let the reverse brainwash begin

So, what are we going to do in this book? How do we proceed?

We're going to de-programme ourselves by talking to psychologists and neuroscientists about the love-hooked messages we get from society, and what goes on in our crazy-in-love brains.

We'll dig around in the messages we get from literature, films and TV, that condition us to be obsessed with romantic love (The *Bridget Jones* trilogy ended with, of course, a wedding). These messages get under our skin, they dig into our subconscious, they make us think that our happy-ever-after has to involve a couple silhouetted against a sunset. Y'know what? It doesn't.

If you do want to date, I'm going to tell you how I learned to do it *moderately*, without turning into a deranged Instagram stalker, and without thinking I was in love with some dude I'd known for two weeks.

Most importantly, we're going to locate and free a spring of single joy. And make sure it never goes away again.

ACKNOWLEDGEMENTS

First up, I am forever indebted to my readers. Without you buying, sharing and recommending my books, I would not be able to continue to do this job that I love so damn much. Your continued support, instagrams, tweets and beautiful emails mean so much to me; I only wish I could splice myself to hang out with/online chat with you all.

Bottomless thanks to my agent Rachel Mills, a thoughtful, bookish yogini who has bucketloads of business verve. An eternal debt also to everyone at Aster and Octopus, particularly my talented firework of a publisher Steph, PR extraordinaire Karen, my lovely 'maximizer' editor Pauline, sales whizz Kevin, digital mastermind Matt, and my patient designer Yasia, who deals with my zany ideas with grace, bears with me when we're on edit 17, and ultimately creates covers I am utterly besotted with.

I could not write these books without the cavernous knowledge of my experts, in this instance Hilda Burke, Dr Alex Korb, Dr Sonja Lyubomirsky, Professor Vybarr Cregan-Reid, Dr Rick Hanson and Dr Michelle Segar. Thank you so much for your time and genius insights. Gratitude also goes out to Charlotte Bowerman who was a tireless, marvellous research assistant, digging up obscure sources – and finding brand new studies I had no idea even existed.

Colossal thanks to my first readers, in no particular order – Kate Faithfull-Williams, Jen Nelson, Andy Mac, Laurie McAllister, Lou Gray, Barbara and Anna Ford. Your feedback and time was invaluable, thank you honeys. Finally, and on a personal level, I feel so incredibly grateful to have such kind, clever and funny friends and family (both biological and step-), with whom I have the most gorgeous, ordinary, homespun moments.